Bag Balm
and Duct Tape

Bag Balm and Duct Tape

Tales of a Vermont Doctor

BEACH CONGER, M.D.

LITTLE, BROWN AND COMPANY
Boston · Toronto · London

FIRST EDITION

Some of these chapters are expanded versions of newspaper articles originally published in *The Valley News*,
West Lebanon, New Hampshire.

Library of Congress Cataloging-in-Publication Data

Conger, Beach, 1941–
    Bag balm and duct tape.
    1. Conger, Beach, 1941–   . 2. Physicians
(General practice)—Vermont—Biography. 3. Medicine,
Rural—Vermont—Anecdotes. 4. Physicians (General
practice)—Vermont—Anecdotes. I. Title.
R154.C553A3   1988   610.92′4 [B]   88-6870

10 9 8 7 6 5 4 3 2

FG

Published simultaneously in Canada
by Little, Brown & Company (Canada) Limited

PRINTED IN THE UNITED STATES OF AMERICA

To the staff at Mt. Ascutney Hospital,
because they put up with me, and to Trine,
because she doesn't

Bag Balm *and* Duct Tape

INTRODUCTION

DEAR READER,

When I told one of my colleagues I was keeping a diary, he said, "What a dumb thing to do." His comment, which, to someone who doesn't understand doctors, might sound rude, did not upset me. I knew he was thinking about the kind of diary that his sister kept, one for recording her most intimate thoughts so that when she was grown up, she could read through it and remember what it was like being young. Hers was the kind of diary that had a little lock and was hidden someplace in her room where nobody could find it — except her brother, who sneaked into her bedroom, found the diary, jimmied it open, and read it, stopping only when he got to the page that said, "Brother, you better stop reading my diary or you are going to be sorry! And I mean it!"

This is not that kind of diary — the kind one keeps for one's own personal pleasure. In fact, it wasn't even my idea to write a diary.

It was my mother's.

I was a very sensitive child. (This may sound suspiciously like an intimate diary remark, but as you will see, it isn't.) I needed large amounts of praise to get through even an ordinary day. My mother did not worry about this at first.

She figured that sensitivity was just one of those stages children go through, and that I would outgrow it. She was a little concerned when she couldn't find anything about the "sensitive child" in her book *The Child from Five to Ten*, the book she read when I had done something that worried her and she needed reassurance that it was normal. She did her best to help me. She tried to protect me from those things that are likely to upset a sensitive child. Like being told to behave myself. Or to mind my own business.

By the time I got to high school, and she was calling up the girls I wanted to ask out so that I wouldn't have to hear them say no, she realized that my tendency toward sensitivity had developed into a definite condition. She knew that something had to be done, or else people would look at me when I was being sensitive and say, "That Beach Conger sure is selfish. I bet his mother spoiled him rotten." She knew that I would be in real trouble if I had to be an ordinary adult. She knew I needed to be the kind of adult whose sensitivity would be respected. So she decided that I should become a doctor.

This turned out to be the perfect solution to my problems.

One day, when I was visiting my mother, she said, "Chip" — she used this intimate form of address only when we were alone; in public she always addressed me as My Son, Doctor Conger — "you ought to write a diary and publish it as a book, so that mothers who have sensitive children can find out about being a doctor. That would be a real public service."

I always follow my mother's advice. So I wrote this diary.

When my patients found out about the diary, they got a little nervous. Patients are very shy. They don't like a lot of publicity about their problems. For example, if Mrs. Jones came into the office because she thought she had pneumonia, and it turned out to be nothing more than a cold, she would be extremely embarrassed if I blabbed this to the whole world.

I talked this problem over with my wife. She listens to everything I say and watches everything I do so that she can tell me when I have gone "over the line," as she puts it. She is Norwegian and a lawyer. She can draw a very fine line.

She said that actual names would definitely be over the line. Furthermore, she thought that fictitious names with actual situations would be very close to the line and at times might have a tendency to wander over to the other side. I didn't want anybody unhappy or anybody, especially myself, in trouble. So I decided to use fictitious names, and the situations I made mostly true, except for a few details that are not really important. This means that anyone who wants to use the book as a source of inspiration can do so without fear of being misled.

One final note. I realize that there are two types of people who will be reading this book: serious readers and sex fiends. To make things easier for the serious readers, who will be referring to the book whenever they have a question about doctoring, I have annotated it. Every time I say something edifying, I preface the observation with the phrase *Serious Reader Note.*

Sex fiends, I am afraid, have no such assistance, so you are just going to have to muddle along until you find what you are looking for.

1

Spring was yielding center stage to summer as I drove north on Route 5. To my right was the Connecticut River, separated from the road by wide strips of fertile farmland, where the dark river-bottom soil sprouted a stubble of new corn. On the left, rising three thousand feet above the valley floor, was a mountain. Its broad, fir-covered back sloped up from the river until it reached a treeless summit.

Four hundred years ago, this land was part of the Algonquin nation. The tribes that inhabited it were fiercely independent and quite possessive about territories. To keep peace, the Algonquins had established a governing council. The council was responsible for resolving intertribal disputes. It was called Abenaki, which means "people of the sunrise."

The first white settlers to arrive were very impressed with how civilized the Indians were. So much so, they decided to name the mountain Abenaki in their honor. The Algonquins never said anything to the white folks about how much they appreciated this tribute. But that doesn't mean they were ungrateful. They moved away shortly after the settlers arrived, and they were so busy packing at the time that they didn't have an opportunity to say thank you.

Geological ages ago, Abenaki Mountain belonged to the Green Mountain clan, but it grew restless for new horizons, and so it emigrated eastward. Although its homeland is easily visible from the top, Abenaki, except for one foothill on its western flank, is a solitary mountain. The foothill isn't much company. Until 1975, when a real estate developer, hoping it would help sell his condominiums, called it Little Abenaki Mountain, it didn't even have a name.

Abenaki is not a great mountain. Its slopes never get quite enough snow, and the splendor of its open summit is diminished by a cluster of transmitting towers, access of which comes from a paved road that runs across its back like a giant scar.

Nonetheless, to those who live beneath, it is a good mountain. Nobody complains when their skis scrape the rocks, or the antennas block their view. It is, after all, their mountain.

Mine too. From now on this valley would be home. The place I would spend my days healing the sick and my nights by the fire. A quiet place, where my worries would not be whether we all could survive a nuclear war, but whether my firewood would last until spring.

Vermont has always been a special place for me. It was not so much the cabin on Lake Bomoseen where we had taken our vacation every summer when I was a child, nor even my hideout in the boulders, where I secreted myself to indulge in heroic boyhood fantasies. No. It wasn't any actual Vermont place that captivated a nostalgic spot in my memory. It was the idea of Vermont. A mysterious, faraway wonderland to get to which, when we went there from our home in Westchester County, we had to drive forever along narrow, winding roads that seemed to lead straight to nowhere, and then, when they got there, kept on going.

This trip in my rented Ford Galaxy had taken three

hours and forty minutes from New York City to the Massachusetts-Vermont border. Partly it was shorter because I had lost my childhood ability to experience every minute of a trip in its entirety. But it wasn't only me. The road too had changed. I-91 bore little resemblance to the road we used to take, a road that meandered about the countryside, stopping at every town it found, so that when it went from Barnet to East Barnet, it did so by way of Barnet Center and Barnet Falls. I-91 is straight and wide. It doesn't stop anywhere. It doesn't even have signs, so you have no idea where the next Howard Johnson's is, or how many baskets are left in Basketville. I-91 is for people in a hurry. People who, when they want to get away from it all, don't want to waste time in the getting part, they just want to get to their destination so they can get right down to the business of relaxing.

I left I-91 at the Massachusetts border and got on Route 5. I was in no hurry. Hurry, after all, was something possessed only by Flatlanders, that ethnic group occupying most of the planet — excepting only a small, somewhat mountainous spot in the northeastern corner of North America — and from which, by virtue of taking up residence in this same spot, I had just resigned.

Route 5 ambled north along the river, stopping at each of the small towns that bordered it — towns that once were thriving vessels on the industrial seas, but now, left awash in the wake of the twentieth century, scrabbled stubbornly just to stay afloat. Brattleboro. Bellows Falls. Rockingham. Dumster.

DUMSTER 5 MILES read the sign. I picked up the letter on the seat next to me and, for the tenth time that day, read it to myself.

> Go past Dumster Vista Apartments to the traffic light. Turn left at the light. About a mile up the

road, just before it turns to dirt, there is another road off to the right which leads into a pasture. The hospital is at the back of the pasture, 200 yards from the road. Look for a big wooden sign with flowers around it. It is hard to miss the sign, but if you do, don't worry, because the road stops a quarter of a mile beyond.

Looking forward to seeing you in July.

> Yours for health,
> Herbert Shiftley, Administrator
> Emmeline Talbot Memorial Hospital

It had started on a Sunday evening. I was sitting in the living room reading the paper when the telephone rang. I wondered whether to get up and answer it — not because I was lazy, but because I was uncertain. My chair was located at a point precisely equidistant between my telephone and my neighbor's, so that I couldn't tell, from my current position, for whom the bell rang. I looked out the window and saw my neighbor. He also was sitting in his living room and happened to be in a chair that had precisely the same acoustical relationship to my phone as his did to mine. We looked at each other. We shared one thought — the thought that, California or not, it was the other person's turn to check the phone.

At the same time that I was downstairs partaking of this metaphysical experience with my neighbor, Trine was upstairs festering in preparation for her midterm law school examinations. She was assisted in her efforts by a drip emanating from the bathroom faucet. The drip happened to be of exactly the same frequency as that with which her brain waves were propagating, so that when the sound passed into her ear, across the tympanic membrane, and into the cochlea, and then ascended the auditory nerve to the occipital cortex, it disrupted the current transmitted between the two hemispheres as they argued over which of them was responsible for rules of evidence. The left claimed priority because the rules were facts, and facts clearly belonged to the left. And the right said that if she was going to need access to these rules in an emotionally stressful situation, it might be a good idea for them to be in the custody of someone who was not likely to fly off the handle.

The drip was particularly disturbing because there was nothing she could do about it. The faucet from which it emanated was not across the hall. It was across the driveway. Trine came down to escape the dripping faucet just as I got up to answer the unringing phone. We met at the foot of the stairs. Relating to each other as we did, we could tell that we were sharing the same feeling — maybe it was time to end our California experience.

It had been a good experience. We had met in Berkeley, in one of the large redwood houses that used to be single-family homes, but now, nuclear families having by and large disintegrated in the Bay Area, were occupied by collectives, intimate clusters of related and unrelated people living in Brownian relationships, where the combinations of related and unrelated changed so frequently and so imperceptibly that nobody noticed until he got up one morning and discovered that, like the passage of fall, all the leaves were gone. So it was no big deal when I found that I had more in common with the Norwegian ski instructor who lived in the front bedroom on the third floor than I did with my wife; while she, the wife, turned out to prefer the company of the sanitary engineer who lived on the sunporch to that of her husband by her present marriage.

Two household members were bothered by this switch. They were Matt and Dylan, the only tangible evidence of our ten-year training marriage. Their initial disfavor, caused by some confusion about lines of parental authority, quickly vanished when they determined that the amount of attention had doubled, whereas the amount of discipline, once they learned to trade it for their affections, actually diminished.

We lived in this blissful state for about six months. Then, late one afternoon, there was a knock on our door. On our porch were two men. They were from the Immigration Service. They asked if we knew anything of the whereabouts of one Treen Bitch. (This appellation arose not from a lack of respect for the person in question, but from their ignorance of Norwegian phonetics. Our resident Scandinavian linguist, not wanting to embarrass them, did not correct their error.) We invited them in for tea, and they told us that the woman in question had been eluding them for over a year by enrolling in various graduate schools and then dropping out just before classes started. We all agreed this was scandalous behavior and promised to keep an eye out for her. After tea they thanked us for being so helpful and left.

An emergency meeting of the house was convened. After much discussion, a plan was devised, voted on, and approved unanimously.

Trine and I would get married.

Which we did. October 18, 1973, in Berkeley City Hall. My brand-new ex-wife gave away the groom, the sanitary engineer was best man, and the kids carried flowers. The event caused quite a stir in Berkeley. For a while nobody would relate to us. Then we explained the whole situation, pointing out that Trine would have been deported if she hadn't married an American, and everybody conceded that getting married under those circumstances was not a cop-out but a rip-off and was therefore right on. They got a little suspicious when we continued to live together after getting married. After Nadya was born, and the three of us, with whichever of the other two kids it was our turn for, moved into a small house of our own, they realized they had been tricked. But by that time it was too late for organized protest.

We had enjoyed Berkeley, but it was time to get on with our life. We sat down in the living room and discussed what we would need in our new place to live. There were five items on our final list:

1. Four seasons
2. No neighboring phones
3. One law school
4. One medical school
5. One Chinese restaurant

The law school was for Trine, who, after not becoming a social worker, a criminologist, or a clinical psychologist, decided what she really wanted to be was a lawyer. The medical school was for me. Up to this point in my career, all my doctoring had been in big medical centers, first Boston, then Atlanta, and finally San Francisco. They provided a very reassuring environment. Whenever I didn't know what to do, help was never more than an "I'll be back in a minute" away. I was not yet ready to practice medicine outside the professional womb.

We examined our needs and studied the maps. One place stood out above all the others: Stowe, Vermont. Shortly after we got married we had stayed there for a week at Christmas, at the Trapp Family Lodge. We had a wonderful time, so we were pretty sure that Stowe would be right for us.

Stowe did not have a medical school or a law school, but it was within commuting distance of Burlington, wherein resided the University of Vermont and Medical Center

Hospital. Trine could transfer to the law school to finish her studies, and I had no doubt that there would be a place for me in the medical center.

We were all set for our scouting trip when Trine got a letter from the University of Vermont. "Dear Ms. Bech," it said. "Thank you for thinking of the University of Vermont, but we don't have a law school. You want Vermont Law School, which is located in South Royalton."

We pulled out the map of Vermont. After considerable searching, we found South Royalton. Its lettering indicated the number of inhabitants to be fewer than two hundred and fifty. Around South Royalton were spaces without any lettering at all. The legend said that these spaces were gores. We had never heard of a gore, so we looked it up in the dictionary. Among the many definitions, only two seemed to fit:

1. dirt, mud
2. a triangular piece of land

This didn't help us much. We went to the library and looked through back issues of *Vermont Life* until we found an article by a New York City stockbroker who had moved to Buel's Gore, where he made his living off the land. The article said that a gore was an unincorporated area that was governed by an overseer. It did not mention any Chinese restaurants.

"We could never live there," I said.

"Don't give up so easily," Trine replied. She took the map and drew a circle around South Royalton. "Look!" she said. "Here's Dartmouth College. It's practically next door." She was quite excited about her discovery.

I was not.

To me, Dartmouth was a place of heathens, a cultural

wilderness inhabited by uncivilized creatures who spent their time drinking beer and abusing women. Not exactly the kind of place a person would want to settle down and raise a family, nor the kind of place one would want to admit working at when it came time to write to one's alumni bulletin. But I couldn't offer any better alternatives, so I swallowed my pride and wrote a letter to Dartmouth Medical School announcing my availability.

Some weeks later I received in the mail an envelope from Dr. Maxwell Stanley, Chairman, Department of Medicine. I opened it, expecting to find within something like "Dear Dr. Conger, We are thrilled that you are interested in joining the Dartmouth-Hitchcock Medical Center. Don't worry about details. We'll work those out when you get here. Yours, Max." This is what I found:

March 17, 1985
Berkshire Medical Group Inc.
47 Ridgeview Drive
Pittsfield, Mass. 01234

Dear Dr. Stanley:
   I am a solo practitioner internist who is looking for a younger partner to join me. If any of your residents might be interested in this opportunity, please have them send me a *curriculum vitae*.

Sincerely yours,
Benjamin Tashman, M.D.

Dr. Stanley was a man who deserved his position. He had killed two birds with no stones.

We thought about giving up the whole idea and moving to Mendocino County. Then one day, while I was listlessly perusing the *New England Journal of Medicine,* I discovered the following adverstisement:

> Excellent opportunity for well-qualified internist to assume practice of retiring general practitioner in small, but fully equipped, community hospital in central Vermont. Superb recreational and cultural facilities nearby. Write Box 26 NEJM.

I wrote to Box 26. It turned out to be Emmeline Talbot Hospital in Dumster, Vermont. One of their general practitioners was retiring after forty years of dedicated service to the community, and they wanted to replace him with a similarly motivated young fellow. As luck would have it, Dumster fell within the circle we had drawn. Although its lettering was not very big, it was at least two grades larger than South Royalton. I sent off my résumé.

A week later I got a call from Mr. Shiftley. He was pleased to tell me that I was just the person they were looking for. Would I be able to start next month?

I was flabbergasted. Didn't they want to meet me? I asked. No, he didn't think that would be necessary. The trustees had checked my credentials, and they were sure I would work out just fine.

Trine and I talked it over. It was rather sudden, but it was our last hope. And they really seemed to want me. Besides, if it didn't work out, we could always leave when Trine finished law school.

I called back the next day and accepted the job.

A faded sign, its message almost obscured by surrounding bushes, informed me that I had reached my destination.

WELCOME TO DUMSTER
HOME OF THE HORNETS

My pulse quickened in anticipation of the first glimpse of my new hometown — a town where I could stroll with my family on a quiet evening, or watch the high school band perform on the Fourth of July; a town where people shared their lives, not in the exhibitionist style of California, but with the quiet respect that was born out of the knowledge that each person's fortunes were inextricably intertwined with everyone else's.

I was greeted at the entrance to the town proper by a huge structure not so much standing as leaning — for *standing* implies an architectural posture that the building had long since lost — on the west side of the street. Rising five stories above the ground and covering what would have been a city block had Dumster been a city, it looked as if it had been airlifted from Brooklyn. It was a genuine tenement.

At the rear, of which view I now partook, was a latticework of crumbling porches that clung to the building like rotting vines. Paint flaked from its walls in such profusion as to create an impression that the edifice was molting. The roof, suffering from a severe case of receding shingles, appeared to be in imminent danger of descending to the street below. Geraniums in distress, calling to be rescued, perched precariously on windowsills.

A freshly painted sign proclaimed the structure to be Dumster Vista Apartments. (This title, as I later learned, was the latest in a series the owners had used to try and change the building's image. It didn't work. Everybody still called it the Block.)

Constructed in the 1920s to house Dumster's factory workers, the Block had aged less gracefully than its original inhabitants, who had long since bought their own homes and moved out, leaving the building to those who stood on a considerably lower rung of the social ladder.

Opposite the Block was a road that led down toward the river. Along it were a factory and an apparently deserted railroad switching yard. Between the railroad tracks and the river was a narrow strip of land consisting primarily of concrete pilings and what looked like, and in fact were, the remnants of houses. In 1933 Acme Tool and Die constructed a row of beautiful homes along the riverbank and offered them at cost to its managers, hoping in this way to entice them to live in Dumster. Riverview Drive was a flourishing community until 1937, when a flood washed away the riverbank.

Dumster did not exactly fit the vision I had of my Vermont hometown. Did the trustees anticipate that this would be the case, and was that the reason for them to hire me sight unseen — unseen not, as I thought, me by them, but rather them by me? It was equally possible that I would not quite match Dumster's vision of the person who would replace the country doctor whom they had loved and respected for the last forty years. Ours was a mail-order marriage, conceived out of necessity. Would it become a relationship sustained by love?

2

SERIOUS READER NOTE: Starts are very important. If something gets off on the right foot, the momentum generated can usually guarantee that, regardless of what obstacles may appear down the road, things will turn out OK.

One situation where a good start is especially crucial is life. If parents and child are relating well to each other as the latter makes his way from womb to world, the next twenty years will pretty much take care of themselves. This is why we now place so much emphasis on how things go during the actual moment of birth, trying to make sure that everything from lighting to seating arrangements is in proper order when the blessed event takes place.

Unfortunately this principle was not always appreciated. People used to consider the delivery of a child to be no big deal. As a result, many an innocent babe was victimized by careless handling when he started his voyage on the sea of life. He was simply plopped in his boat and allowed to drift off without so much as a shove to get him headed in the right direction, and certainly without a crowd on the dock to cheer him on. As a result, when he finally figured out what was going on, he was out on the open sea, with not the faintest idea where he was, and he had to spend the rest of his life trying to find the right course.

A day is like a life, only on a smaller scale. The course of a day gets fixed pretty early in its existence. Even before breakfast. Not that breakfast is unimportant: a bad breakfast can ruin an otherwise auspicious day, and a good one can really help it keep up the pace. But it can't salvage a day that has already gone astray. The critical time for establishing a good day is not when a person sits down at the breakfast table. It is when he gets out of bed.

Take today, for example. Because it was the first day for my diary, I wanted it to be just right. I planned to get up early, go for a brisk run in the cool morning air, take a long, hot shower, and then sit down to a hearty breakfast of granola, English muffins, and a pot of Twining's Earl Grey tea served in my favorite teacup — a teacup that has on it a lovely blue castle surrounded by beautiful blue trees, under which a blue prince and princess stroll happily on their blue lawn.

The night before, I laid out my running clothes in proper order, put a glass of orange juice on the table for a quick carbo load, and set the alarm for five-thirty. I would have preferred to use my clock radio so that I could set it to WVPR and be awakened by the mellow sounds of classical music, but public radio does not get up until six. I was using instead the windup alarm clock my mother had given me as a high school graduation present, explaining as she did that, of all the things she had done for me that I would never fully appreciate, but without which my life would have been a much greater struggle than I could possibly imagine, the clock would do the one thing that was more important and less appreciated than all the others.

I called the clock Mom in honor of this speech. Mom was not like the modern clocks that stop at every minute, so that if you awaken in the middle of the night because of a bad dream you know it occurred at 3:07 A.M. Mom was an express model: sleep time and wake-up time. That was it. In recent years I hadn't used Mom much, but I kept her on hand for occasions when I wanted to be sure I would get up. I went to bed knowing that everything was in order for a perfect day.

I was awakened by a scream so shrill, I was sure it came from either the smoke detector or my daughter.

It was Mom.

Whether I had just grown unaccustomed to her voice, or whether Mom was releasing pent-up hostility, the sound penetrated my brain like the whine of a dentist's drill. I stumbled out of bed. I looked at my running uniform. I looked out the window at a gray, drizzling morning. I knew that running was not going to get this day back on the right track.

I needed a pill.

I bolted for the bathroom and flung open the medicine-cabinet door. There was a jar of Vicks VapoRub, some broken Q-tips, and a rusty pair of tweezers. But none of my pretty little bottles. They had been thrown out when we moved, and I had not yet had time to replenish my stock.

I was about to head for the refrigerator, intending to satisfy my medicinal needs with the remnants of Sunday's batch of fudge brownies, when my eye was attracted by an object partially concealed by some dirty Kleenex. It was a pill bottle. I pulled it out into the light.

I read the label with disbelief. How many times — in trying to lessen the guilt of distraught parents who had just discovered one of their children using drugs — had I said "It can happen to anyone"? I couldn't begin to count. But never for a moment did I think that one day, one of those anyones could be me. There could be no doubt, however, whose bottle this was. Its proximity to an uncapped tube of Clearasil was proof enough.

What a fool I had been: so involved in being important that I had neglected to be a parent. Too busy as Doctor

Conger to be Daddy Beach. And when he really needed his father, the one person who could have given him what he needed, his father wasn't there. He turned elsewhere, to the pharmacological terrorist that, masquerading as a harmless nutritional supplement, sabotages a physician's most basic power, the power of the prescription.

ASCORBIC ACID

It is not that vitamin C does anyone any good that makes it anathema to doctors. The threat stems from an infinitely more dangerous quality of the drug: it does no harm.

My hand frozen on the bottle, I stood there for what seemed like an eternity. Then, before I knew what I was doing, I took one. A second. A third. Down the hatch they went, all fifty pills.

I was at the end of Maple Street when my stomach began to complain. It had no intention of going through its first day on a new job with no more sustenance than the equivalent of eight gallons of orange juice. Hoping that I would be able to quiet this gastric protest with something from the hospital cafeteria, I turned right and started up the hill toward the hospital. I had only gone a few steps when I had to stop. Propelled by some invisible force, I turned and headed in the opposite direction. At first it was only an indistinct glow. Drawing closer, I could see that the light came from a sign. As I reached Main Street the letters burned through the morning fog.

NAT'S LUNCH

With some trepidation, for Nat's did not look like the kind of eating establishment that catered to my customary breakfast menu, I entered the establishment. A single glance was enough to confirm my fears. If Nat's fare was like its clientele, its offerings would be more substantial than those to which I was accustomed. They were. Nat favored fat over fiber and grease over granola. The cholesterol content of an average meal at Nat's exceeded the annual consumption by a Krishna commune. Nat's was a nutritional den of iniquity.

I sat down at the counter. In front of me was a huge stack of Nat's *specialité de la maison*, Chocolate-Covered Jelly Donuts Under Glass. "Feed me!" demanded my stomach. I grabbed two of the largest and gulped them down while I waited for my order, a Hunter's Breakfast: three fried eggs, two sausage patties, a big pile of hash browns, and a generous covering of maple syrup. It was good. And relaxing. Very relaxing. My newspaper became too heavy to hold. I put it down on the counter, my head alongside it. It was some time before I could pick it up again.

CONGER COPS NOBEL NOD

STOCKHOLM (AP) Beach Conger, the country doctor from Dumster, Vermont, who discovered that massive doses of vitamin C taken immediately before a cholesterol-rich meal could block the formation of atherosclerotic plaques, received medicine's highest honor today. In a typically modest statement, Conger said of his work, which has virtually eliminated the need for dietary restrictions in the prevention of heart disease and strokes, "It was no big deal."

Health professionals around the world were much less restrained in their assessment of Conger's work. Olaf Pedersen, chairman of the Nobel Prize committee, hailed the discovery as "the greatest breakthrough since the invention of the artificial egg." Kitty Ritzel, president of the American Heart Association, said it was "really neat" and announced plans to make April Vitamin C Month. The Citrus Growers Association and the National Dairy Council both have named Conger their Man of the Year.

Although it is still unclear exactly how vitamin C works to prevent atherosclerosis, . . .

My dream was ended abruptly by an urgent call from my stomach telling me that it had just figured out how vitamin C protects the body against cholesterol. It suggested we discuss its findings in private. I rushed to the bathroom. There I threw up my breakfast. Then I threw up fifty partially digested pills.

By the time I had cleaned myself up and gotten to the hospital, it was nine o'clock. I walked briskly through the crowded waiting room, hoping that no one would notice that I resembled the survivor of a weekend drinking binge more than a doctor coming to work. I entered my new office and closed the door. Before I could compose myself, the door opened and in walked Margaret Stone. Mrs. Stone was a small but solid woman in her early fifties. Her black hair was heavily stippled with streaks of gray, and her face looked as if, under the proper circumstances, it might be kind. At present it was impassive.

SERIOUS READER NOTE: Doctors, as I mentioned in the introduction, have difficulty functioning as normal adults. It is important, therefore, that each of us be under the care of someone who can ensure that we get through each day without being criticized for something that, if an ordinary adult did it, would be considered rude or inconsiderate — such as missing an appointment or going off to tea while a patient was waiting to be examined. This is why every doctor is supervised by a responsible person.

———————◄•►———————

Mrs. Stone had raised five children, trained two husbands (Her first, whom she had spent ten of the best years of her life getting into reasonable shape, ran off with a woman he met in the Laundromat. Mrs. Stone took no chances with the second. Before she remarried, she bought a washer and a dryer.), and been in charge of Old Doc Franklin for twenty-eight years. Mrs. Stone was a very responsible person.

"Good morning, Mrs. Stone," I said, trying to sound authoritative as I introduced myself to her. "What is on our schedule today?"

"My name is Maggie," she replied. "Mr. Purlife is on your schedule. Has been for the last hour." She finished speaking but remained at the door, not so much waiting as studying, trying to decide whether I was a younger version of her beloved Dr. Franklin or a whippersnapper. Her opinion seemed to be inclining toward the latter.

This was hardly an auspicious beginning for my new career. Maggie was Dumster's weathervane for which way the wind blew on the new doctor. The slightest qualification to her praise, the slightest hesitation in her voice —anything less than total and abject admiration — could spell my doom.

What to do? I could make an excuse. Maggie did not look like someone who took well to excuses. I could tell the truth and put myself at her mercy. She seemed the forgiving type — but I couldn't be sure. There was one other option.

"Fine. Tell him I'll be there in a minute. I have to review his chart before I can examine him."

"Very well." She turned to leave. At the door she stopped and said, "Welcome to Dumster."

I had been accepted. Not because I deserved it, but because Maggie recognized that I was not at fault. I couldn't help it. I was a doctor.

I thumbed through Mr. Purlife's chart, but I couldn't concentrate on the words. I wasn't worried about what might be ailing him. I didn't know if I would even be able to talk to him. In California, I related to my patients, or I saw where they were coming from, or maybe shared their space. Office visits involved a lot of nonverbal communication, especially hugging, but not much actual talking. From what I had heard about Vermonters, they would be pretty good at the nonverbal, but not much into hugging.

I had spent the past week reviewing my medical school notes on how to take a history. I practiced asking the kind of questions doctors were supposed to ask and writing down the answers, as if they were important in solving the problem at hand. And just in case I got nervous when the time came, I had memorized my opening lines, the way I used to do before I went out on a date:

"Good morning, Mr. ————. Some weather we're having. You are my first patient in Dumster, but I have seen many other patients in California and Georgia and Boston. I am going to ask you some questions. Some of them may seem difficult. Don't worry. Just answer them the best you can, and everything will be fine."

On first impression, Harold Purlife was not a very remarkable person. Second and third impressions confirmed the first. He was a tall, thin man and had a slight kyphosis to his thoracic spine, so that when standing he resembled a piece of spaghetti that had been thrown against the wall to see if it was cooked. His only truly distinguishing feature was his forehead. It was a great board, large and square and, except for one deep groove traversing its entire length, completely flat. When the forehead was in doubt — which, judging from the depth of the groove, I would say was often — it opened into a giant crevasse into whose depths it looked as if his whole upper body, face, neck, and chest would fall. This physiognomic wonder was the result of many years of poring over figures that the forehead, being of a suspicious nature, was never quite able to trust. The forehead worked at Acme, where Mr. Purlife was the chief accountant. For thirty-five years he had worked in the same building at the same desk. He graduated from Dumster High School in 1943 and, after the draft board declared him 4F because of his eyesight, went to accounting school in Boston. He went straight from school to Acme, where he contributed to the war effort by making sure that Acme didn't overcharge the Defense Department for the ball bearings it made. He was fifty-nine years old, and he lived with his eighty-five-year-old mother in an old brick house on North Main Street.

If Harold Purlife did not seem the kind of patient with whom I would be able, years later, to reminisce about our meeting, at least he was harmless. I congratulated him on the honor of being my first patient, gave my little speech, and got down to business.

SERIOUS READER NOTE: Asking questions is a very tricky part of the doctor-patient relationship. The doctor needs to ask questions in order to obtain vital information, but at the same time does not want to provide an opportunity for the patient to get too talkative, thereby getting into a situation where the doctor might lose control of the conversation. Once a doctor and a patient get to know each other this problem usually disappears, because they have both learned those questions and answers that might get their relationship into trouble and can avoid them.

But at first meeting, a doctor does not know whether his patient might be a gabber, and he has no idea about areas where the patient may be particularly sensitive. So he has to be very careful. This being my first patient, I decided to start conservatively.

———————◄ ♦ ►———————

"Well, Mr. Purlife," I said. "How are you doing?"

Ordinarily, this is a safe opener. Most people, even in a doctor's office, realize that the question has nothing to do with how a person actually feels. They know that the correct answer, regardless of how miserable they might be, is "fine." I waited for Harold Purlife to say "fine" and got ready for my next question, which had to do with whether or not he had ever been exposed to ionizing radiation in his childhood. This is a hard-hitting question, and it never fails to make patients feel that I am really going to find out what is going on.

Mr. Purlife did not say "fine." Instead, he started with an analysis of the relationship between his fiber intake and his current sense of self-worth. Then he described how much his masculinity had improved since he had doubled his vitamin E intake. Too late, I realized that asking Harold Purlife how he felt was like asking him to discuss the meaning of life. He was what people would call a health nut — although it wasn't being healthy he was nutty about, it was working on being healthy.

As he continued with an explanation of how he was countering the toxicity of food additives through zinc supplements, it became apparent that he knew a lot about nutrition. Some of it might even be true. I certainly couldn't tell. Like any respectable doctor, I knew virtually nothing about vitamins.

It was obvious that Mr. Purlife could continue his monologue indefinitely. I had to cut him off.

"What brings you here today?"

"My metabolism is out of whack."

Things were going from bad to worse. Normal patients recognize that it is their responsibility to provide information that will allow me to make a diagnosis, after which they will listen quietly while I outline a course of action. Normal patients complain of things like tummy pain or trouble breathing or feeling low, symptoms that give me plenty of diagnostic elbow room. But not metabolism. I had no idea what defective metabolism was.

Fortunately, I am well trained to conceal ignorance. From my vast repertoire of probing questions, which give the appearance of gathering vital information but are primarily designed to buy time until I can figure out what to do next, I picked one at random.

"How long has this metabolism problem been going on?"

"Since last Tuesday. Inadvertently, I drank some tea out of Mother's cup. I only use honey, of course, but she puts sugar in hers. I took a ginseng purge right away, but it didn't help. I still feel run-down. I'm afraid that the sugar must have gummed up something in my system."

By this time I was pretty sure I knew what Harold Purlife's problem was. I asked him two more questions to make sure.

"Have you taken any medicine for your problem?"

"Heck, no. I don't take chemicals. Only the purest ingredients in this body." He tapped himself proudly on the chest. "I want to keep it in top running order."

"How about vitamins?"

"Vitamins? Naturally. Couldn't do without them. Therapeutic Totals, Super E, B Complex Multiform, high-potency zinc, lecithin — I take a double dose; can't take any chances at my age — and C, of course. Two thousand milligrams a day." He paused for a minute. "I see what you're getting at. You think maybe I'm not getting enough C. Maybe I should boost it up to four thousand milligrams until things straighten out?"

It was just as I suspected. Harold Purlife was suffering from vitamania.

———— ◆ ————

Serious Reader Note: Vitamania used to be a disease found only among poppers. Nobody knows what causes a person to turn into a popper, but the telltale signs — neat arrays of bottles at the breakfast table, orderly consumption of each pill at its appointed time, panic when supplies are low — often appear shortly after someone has been in a hospital. This has led some researchers to speculate that it may be caused by a germ or toxic substance that resides in medical institutions and attacks people when their resistance is down.

For a popper, the value of a pill depends more on how it looks than on any medicinal effect it may have. Therefore, the colors and shapes of pills are far more important than their contents. When drug companies, in an effort to sell more vitamins, spiffed them up by replacing the standard dull brown with bright blues and bold reds, and added innovative oblongs and pentagons to the traditional flat round, poppers got turned on to vitamins. They switched from drugstores to health-food stores. They discovered that not only were vitamins cheaper and prettier than what the doctor ordered, they were also safer.

Vitamaniacs talked to their friends and relatives about the wonders of vitamins. This got the friends and relatives to thinking, because, while to the outside world friends and relatives always seem to be in pretty good shape, late at night, in the privacy of their own beds, they are festering. They fester about things that seem so insignificant, they would be too embarrassed to mention them to anyone, especially a doctor, but that feel as if they have the potential to turn into something terrible. Things like a pimple in a private place, or a pain in the earlobe. Things that are never mentioned in the pamphlets that list The Warning Signs, and they don't know if it's because the diseases that cause them are too terrifying to mention, or because they are completely unimportant.

So friends and relatives said to themselves, "Why not?" And they went to the store and waited until no one else was around and asked for a bottle of Magnavit Super Grow, "for my wife." Pretty soon everyone was taking vitamins.

Vitamins, because they do not treat any particular illness, are useful not only to people with secret problems, but also as general restoratives. People can take vitamins to be smarter, or sexier, or to fight depression. People can even take vitamins to help them express their feelings.

Harold Purlife was taking vitamins as an expression of moral outrage. He was furious with civilization for all the poisons it had put in the air he breathed, the water he drank, and the food he ate. He took vitamins to purify himself. Not chemical vitamins from pharmaceutical companies. Natural vitamins, from rosehips and oyster shells and bee pollen.

Patients who take natural vitamins are especially difficult to manage. Hanging around health-food stores, they hear a lot of talk about health. Not the kind that begins, "Dr.

Conger is so wonderful. I went to see him last week, and he fixed my . . ." Instead it sounds more like "I went to this doctor, and she said I would need an operation, but I started taking alfalfa and now I feel fine." Such talk tends to foster a poor attitude and a lack of respect for doctors.

I may not know much about vitamins, but I do know how to straighten out a patient with a poor attitude.

"Get on the table."

Startled by my tone, Mr. Purlife quickly complied.

"Open your mouth."

He opened his mouth. I looked inside.

"Hmmmm." I repeated it for emphasis. "Hmmmm."

"Something wrong?" he asked nervously.

"Noticed anything unusual about your urine?"

"What do you mean?" Harold Purlife started to sweat. People who are into health spend a lot of time noticing their excretions. They consider them to be body barometers.

"Any change in color, or perhaps a new odor?"

"Well, last week it was slightly orange. And yesterday it smelled like moldy bread. Does that mean anything?"

"It sounds to me like a mild case of vitamin C poisoning."

"Vitamin C? Poisoning? Impossible! I only take organic C."

"Your poor cells don't care where it comes from, Harold. All they know is that it hurts."

"Come off it, Doc. You're putting me on. They told me doctors would be like this." Harry struck a pose he hoped would pass for defiance.

I wasn't fooled. "It's all a matter of basic trust. Your body is a precision machine, each part constructed to complement the others. Your brain picks out the right foods for you to eat. Your intestinal tract absorbs what you need and gets rid of the rest. Your liver turns the raw materials into useful nutrients. Your bloodstream carries them to the outlying organ. There each cell takes just what it needs, gives back its leftovers, and then uses what it has selected to perform its assigned task. Everything works together in perfect harmony.

"And then you spoil it all by dumping a big load of vitamins down the chute. How do you think that makes your body feel? I'll tell you how: the same way you would feel if you came to work one morning and found some guy from New York City sitting at your desk, brought in by your boss to check on your work. Trust your body, Harry. Trust nature."

"You mean I should get rid of my vitamins?"

"Every last one. Believe me, it's the only way."

"But what about all the pesticides and the preservatives?"

"Two wrongs don't make a right."

"But if I can't take vitamins, what am I going to do to protect my health?"

"That's my job, Harry. We'll start by scheduling you to come in next month for a complete physical."

"I didn't think doctors wanted to bother with healthy people. It's nice to know there's someone who is as interested in me when I'm well as when I'm sick."

"Times have changed, Harry. Think of me as the maintenance man for your body. I'll keep you in good running order — just as long as you check in on a regular basis."

"You can count on that."

3

Times certainly have changed. It wasn't too many years ago that the last thing in the world doctors wanted cluttering up their waiting rooms was healthy people. They had their hands pretty full with the sick ones, riding all over the countryside to visit them and then sitting by their bedside for hours on end when they got there. It may not have been a very efficient way to dispense medical care, but it was excellent public relations, which was very important, because what doctors had to offer in the way of improving a patient's lot in life was pretty skimpy.

Those were the good old days, when people were men, and doctors were gods. Such was Doc Franklin, who, fresh out of medical school, moved to Dumster in 1937 with his old, beat-up Model T and his new, barely broken-in wife. It was right in the middle of the Depression, and people were short enough on cash for things like food and shelter that when it came to paying the doctor, it didn't. His first few years in Dumster, Doc Franklin made ends meet by playing the fiddle at square dances and by selling Mrs. Doc Franklin's Elixir. When doctoring finally started to pay off, he was able to stop the fiddling, but every time he tried to get out of the elixir business, his patients complained so loudly that his wife had to resume production. I hadn't been in town a week when someone came in asking for it. When I told her I didn't have any, she said if I was half the doctor Doc Franklin was — which, by the looks of it, she doubted I was — I would find out how to make it pretty damn quick. The next time I saw Doc Franklin, I asked him what was in it.

"Honey and lemon."

"That's all?"

"Yup."

"Hard to believe people would have so much faith in something as simple as that."

"Isn't it, though. My wife felt the same way. She said it wasn't the honey and lemon at all."

"More like the magic touch of a caring doctor?"

"Something like that. And what we mixed it in."

"What was that?"

"Rupert Bugbee's corn liquor."

Even without the assistance of Rupert's still, when it came to medicine, Doc Franklin was a master at getting a lot from not very much. He had to be. Most of the drugs he had were poisons. Most of the tests he could perform were useless. And most of his knowledge was wrong. All he really had going for him was Doc Franklin. But that was enough — that and a little medicinal sleight of hand. Like the elixir and his famous Green Pills. I learned about the pills from Aaron Penstock, when he threw his back out.

"How did you hurt it?"

"Lifting hay."

"How long ago?"

"Not long."

"Have you ever hurt it before?"

"Yup."

"When?"

"Long time ago."

"What did you do about it?"

"Came here."

"I see. I'd like you to get undressed so I can examine your back."

"No need to."

"I can't treat you without an examination."

"Doc Franklin did."

"I am not Doc Franklin."

"I noticed."

"Well, then, if you don't want an examination, what do you want?"

"Green Pills."

"What's their name?"

"Ain't got no name but Green Pills. Listen, Doc, I didn't come here to fool around. I come here for Green Pills. If you don't know what they is, ask Maggie. She can tell you."

I went to Maggie and asked her if she knew about some kind of green pill that Doc Franklin used to prescribe. She smiled and said yes, they were called Duradyne. I had never heard of Duradyne, so I looked it up in the *Physicians' Desk Reference* for prescription drugs. The *PDR* told me that Duradyne contained a combination of three hundred and twenty-five milligrams of acetylsalicylic acid and sixty milligrams of caffeine. One Duradyne tablet was the pharmacological equivalent of an aspirin and a cup of coffee. I knew better than to tell Mr. Penstock this, so I wrote out a prescription for Duradyne and gave it to him. He looked a little surprised, but he took the prescription without comment. I felt quite pleased with myself at how rapidly I was adapting to country practice.

About twenty minutes later I got a call from Al Marcup, owner and proprietor of Marcup's Drug.

"Hey, Doc," he said. "Penstock just brought me a prescription for Duradyne."

"That's right. I just wrote him one."

"What do you want me to do with it?"

"Why, fill it, of course."

"I don't carry Duradyne."

"Well, then, send him to someone who does."

"That's you."

"Me?"

"Yeah, you. Unless Doc Franklin took them when he retired, you must have a ton of 'em up there."

"You mean he used to fill his own prescriptions?"

"For Green Pills, he did. You see, you don't write a prescription for Green Pills. You put two of 'em in a little brown envelope. You tell the patient to take one when he gets home and another one two hours later. Then you warn him that if things aren't better in four hours, it could be something serious, and you might have to send him to Hanover."

"I see. Well, thanks for the information."

"No trouble, Doc. Always glad to help you young fellows out. Especially now that Doc Franklin's gone."

He was right. I never could have gotten through the first few weeks without Doc Franklin's help — not that I actually asked his advice about anything, but just being able to say, when a patient questioned my recommendations, that I had checked it out with Doc Franklin got me out of a lot of tight spots. Unfortunately, he died just one month after I arrived. Dropped dead while fishing. The coroner put down heart attack as the cause of death, but everybody knew that wasn't it. The heart attack just happened to be the most convenient way for him to get rid of the carcass of a life that had ended when he stopped working. What killed him was retirement.

Doc Franklin was always there, and he was always comforting. People said that healing powers radiated from him like the heat of a woodstove, so that all he had to do was walk into the room and a person felt better. Especially the women. Muriel Blackington had terrible arthritis. I remember the first time she came to see me, and I asked to take a look at her joints. She held out her hands. I took them the way I might a surgical instrument, inspected them, and then gave them back.

"Your hands don't look too bad," I said. "Let's take a look at your knees."

"No," she said quietly.

"I can't help you if I can't examine you," I replied, trying not to show my irritation. It was now my second month in Dumster, and the regular rebuffs I was receiving at my proposals to perform proper examinations were beginning to get on my nerves.

Mrs. Blackington held out her hands again.

"That won't be necessary," I said. "I've seen all I need to know about your hands. What I need to see is the rest of your joints. That way I can better assess the severity of your arthritis."

She took my hands and put them in her gnarled ones. "Looking don't do 'em any good," she said. "Holding is what they want."

We sat there for a few minutes, our hands clasped awkwardly. Then she withdrew and stood up. "If you want to doctor in Dumster, you gotta learn to hold. That was Doc Franklin's way." Without another word, she left.

It was the way of a lot of physicians like Doc Franklin, the ones who had learned to rely mainly on the art of medicine because, for most of their careers, science hadn't been much help. The Good Old Docs. Doctors who practiced healing by intent, which they had acquired not by some conscious effort on their part but by having it given to them by the same patients on whom they would use it. This may have been a little convoluted, but it was the only way it could work, for it was necessary back then, to the well-being of both patient and doctor, that the healing powers, which actually reside in the one being treated, be ascribed to the one offering the treatment.

Doc Franklin had been quite a doctor. There was hardly a person in Dumster who didn't have a story to tell about how wonderful he was. Some of them were even true. When he retired, the town was greatly saddened. So was Doc Franklin.

There are people who are so clever at doing a particular thing very well that as they progress through life, they wind up doing that thing more and more to the exclusion of everything else. And then, when they get to a point where they can't do it anymore and are called upon to do something quite different, which everyone expects them to do just as well, they make a complete mess of it and fall flat on their face. Because it turns out that the first thing was all they were good for.

So it was with Doc Franklin. For fifty years he had been a Good Old Doc — one of the best — from the time he got up early in the morning until he dragged himself into bed late at night. On the rare occasion when he had tried being a person, he had been a dismal failure. His generous, compassionate personality would turn moody and irascible as he struggled unsuccessfully to cope with things that he never had to use as a Good Old Doc. Things like patience, courtesy, and humility. It will come as no surprise to learn that his retirement was hell. Having been Doc Franklin for so long, he just couldn't make a go of it as Walter. He was miserable. His wife was miserable. The whole town was miserable. It was painful to watch, this great doctor turned into such a little man. So when his coronaries mercifully shut down and brought the whole debacle to an end, everybody was more relieved than they would admit.

4

In years gone by, Good Old Docs were plentiful. You could find at least one in every small town. But when science was introduced into the medical waters, their reproductive abilities were irrevocably damaged, so that one by one, as Good Old Docs retired or died off, they were replaced not by one of their own, but by a new breed of doctor: Smart Young Whippersnappers. Smart Young Whippersnappers were very different from their predecessors. They were efficient, scientific, and expensive. They knew the value of a pill — and the value of a buck.

With this new breed of doctor came a new breed of patient, people who were no longer content to sit in a waiting room for hours on end just so they could shell out their hard-earned money on a few pills and platitudes. They wanted service, and they wanted it pronto. When they didn't get it, they complained. "We need more doctors," they said.

The medical profession, recognizing that an excess of doctors diluted not only the quality of medical care but also the quantity of doctors' incomes, was reluctant to accede to these demands. But the politicians were not. "If the people want more doctors, we'll give them more doctors," they replied. They passed a law that provided low-interest loans to students who wanted to study medicine.

This caused quite a stir in medical schools. Even at Harvard. "We know there are plenty of doctors to go around," they said, "but Anyplace Medical School has just doubled its enrollment, and if we have to have more doctors, they should at least be properly trained, properly versed in medical traditions, and know how to tie their tie."

Meanwhile, over at Anyplace a similar discussion was taking place. "We can't sit by while those jerks over at Harvard multiply like rabbits and populate the land with snobs who think that every patient owes them a living. We owe it to the people to train doctors who have compassion for their patients."

All over the country deans sat down with their faculty and came to the same conclusion: we may not need more doctors, but if we are going to have them, they should be ours. Before anybody knew what was happening, a doctor boom was born, and doctors sprouted like crabgrass. Unfortunately, this increase in the number of practicing physicians was not accompanied by a commensurate increase in the number of patients. A lot of doctors wound up sitting around with time on their hands. As you might expect of intelligent people placed in such a situation, we started thinking. We thought about all the people who, just because there was nothing wrong with them, were not getting the benefit of our services or the chance to pay our fees. Having done so much for the ill, was it fair to deny our skills to the well? Had we been a bit hasty in our disregard of the unsick?

Not that the Good Old Docs had completely ignored the healthy. Doc Franklin did his share of "checkouts," as he called them. But Doc Franklin was too busy to waste time with people who didn't need a pill or an operation. This was a Doc Franklin checkout:

DOC FRANKLIN: How do you feel?
PATIENT: I feel OK.
DOC FRANKLIN: You look OK.

We thought especially long and hard about the Doc Franklin–style checkup. It was one of medicine's time-honored traditions, and it had stood us in good stead since the days of Hippocrates. But now, viewed from our new perspective, it did look rather skimpy. After all, how would someone feel if he brought his car in for a checkup and the mechanic said, "Sounds OK to me." So we beefed up the exam. Check the pump pressure. Look for sludge in the gas line. Test the wiring. Inspect the exhaust system. It was a whole new ballgame. We even changed the name: health maintenance, we called it. Healthy people came in. Healthy people went out. We took the credit. It was easy. And it was successful. It was so successful, in fact, that a whole new medical specialty emerged that concentrated on treatment of the well: family practice. Smart Young Whippersnappers flocked to family practice, and people who had never dreamed of becoming patients flocked to their offices.

Medical research soon followed the lead of practitioners. Researchers switched their interest from what caused diseases to what kept them away. They found one factor that stood out above all the others. They determined that if people had this factor, they probably didn't need a doctor, and if they didn't, seeing one wouldn't help. The factor was luck. Fortunately, this research was published before reporters began reading medical journals. Otherwise health maintenance would have been nipped in the bud.

————◄•►————

SERIOUS READER NOTE: I should say right now, since this diary is intended to be of an inspirational nature, that I am not implying that there is absolutely nothing people can do to fend off illness. But for those who don't smoke or make pigs of themselves, the pickings are pretty slim: blood-pressure checks, Pap smears, and mammograms. Everything else is likely to cause more trouble than it is worth. At best a health-maintenance exam shows nothing. At worst it shows that health is little more than an illusion produced by the inability to find illness. It also increases insurance rates.

––––––◄•►–––––

There was no point in explaining all this to Harry Purlife when he came back to see me. It would just complicate things for him, and he was already nervous enough —which is understandable. Health maintenance is a game played with a stacked deck. It starts with the patient in good health. He has to defend his health. I try to destroy it. He has little with which to defend himself against my arsenal of disease-seeking missiles. And even if he is lucky enough to win a game or two, it doesn't matter, because we keep playing until I win for good. Besides, I sell the tickets.

I usually warm up with a "review of systems." This exercise consists of a series of questions directed at how the patient is currently feeling. I may ask him about pains in his chest, or what he thinks of his job, or how often he makes love. I can ask him anything I want, and he must answer truthfully. Otherwise he is not trusting his doctor. The questions create an impression that I am looking for particular problems that may need addressing, but, in fact, the answers are unimportant. Their sole purpose is to put the patient off balance. Such a patient is much more susceptible to accepting the possibility of illness than one who is relaxed and confident. Everybody has some special worry. Since I had already found Harry's, I went straight to it.

"How's that odor doing?"

"What odor?"

Harry's feigned ignorance didn't fool me. He knew perfectly well what odor. Chances were, he had been thinking of nothing else since the last visit. That was OK. If he wanted to volley a bit before I put him away, I was in no hurry.

"I thought you mentioned last month that your urine smelled like moldy bread. Guess I mixed you up with someone else. Sorry about that. Anyway, it's just as well I was wrong."

"That's all right, Doc. With all the patients you have, it must be hard to keep them straight — Wait a minute." Harry pursed his lips while he sipped a little memory refresher. "Of course. How stupid of me to forget. That odor. It's all gone. Don't think it was anything to bother with." He paused to lick his lips. Apparently the refresher hadn't relieved a sudden dryness in his mouth. "Do you?"

"It's not what I think that matters, Harry, unless you want a philosopher for a doctor."

Without further prompting, Harry took off his clothes and jumped up on the examining table.

I looked in his ears. I thumped on his chest. I listened to his heart. Then I tapped on his back, just below the ribs. Harry moved. It was barely perceptible, but I felt it. And Harry felt it. I tapped a little harder. Harry flinched.

"Does that hurt?"

"Nothing I can't stand."

"I am not questioning your toughness. I merely want to know if you have any discomfort that might indicate a problem."

"It's my kidneys, isn't it?"

"It is in the region of the kidneys, yes. But it would be premature to make a diagnosis based on such preliminary information. I will need to do some tests."

"Do you think it's serious?"

"I warned you, Harry. No thinking in here."

"I know. I know. But just tell me one thing. Does it feel like cancer?"

"Suppose I said no. Would that make any difference?"

Harry shook his head. I made him an appointment for the following week and sent him off to the laboratory for an SMA-30. An SMA-30 is a series of thirty blood tests performed by a machine called an auto analyzer. The auto analyzer has done for health maintenance what the cotton gin did for the industrial revolution. It can test everything from cholesterol to magnesium. It is fast, accurate, and cheap. At twenty-five dollars a shot, it is one of the great bargains in medicine.

For me, that is. Using an SMA-30 in health maintenance is like using a net to catch fish. You can't be sure exactly what you'll find, but you'll never come up empty. In Harry's case it was a calcium: 10.5, just barely above the normal limits. It wasn't much, but it was all I needed. I called Harry and gave him the news. I explained to him how important the kidneys were in the regulation of calcium metabolism. I also told him that, although it was very unlikely that a calcium level of 10.5 would be caused by cancer, I couldn't be sure. I would have to order more tests. An intravenous pyelogram, a bone scan, a serum parathormone assay, and a urine immunoelectrophoresis. The urine test alone was one hundred and fifty dollars. "We had to send it to California," I told Harry when he asked about the cost, "in dry ice."

Everything turned out normal. Even his calcium, which had fallen to 9.8.

"So how come my calcium was up?" Harry asked.

"That's a good question. You could have normocalcemic primary hyperparathyroidism. But I suspect you're just a deviation from the norm."

"You calling me a pervert?"

"Not at all. Deviation from the norm is not a moral principle, Harry. It's a statistical one. Whenever a new test is developed, a range is established for normal values. This is done by running the test on a bunch of healthy people. Most of them will have values that fall within rather narrow limits. A few will be higher than the others, and a few lower. Those are the ones we call deviations from the norm. It doesn't mean there's anything wrong with you. It just means you're different. Like being seven feet tall. Or having red hair."

———————————◆▸▬————————————

SERIOUS READER NOTE: Statistics used to be one of those boring subjects that brought upon doctors an overwhelming desire to lie down and take a nap. Only with the advent of health maintenance has its importance to our profession been appreciated. Now it proudly takes a place alongside anatomy and physiology as one of the cornerstones of modern medicine. Especially useful are its concepts "deviation from the norm," "Bayesian probability," and "regression to the mean."

Bayesian probability guarantees that if you order enough tests on a person, at least one of them will be abnormal, even if nothing is wrong. This is very helpful in keeping patients interested in their health-maintenance examinations. Patients who have nothing but normal results tend to forget to come back.

Regression to the mean says that if you repeat a test that is abnormal by Bayesian probability, it will probably be normal. This ensures that every health-maintenance examination has a happy ending — which is also very important, because patients get demoralized if a doctor finds something she can't do anything about, and then they get to thinking that further evaluations would be pointless.

———————————◆▸▬————————————

5

Vermont has two types of towns: radiant and linear.

Radiant towns are easily recognized by their trademark, the town common, a small plot of grass that is the rural equivalent of a vacant lot. From the common radiates, and hence comes the name, an assortment of roads. The public institutions, businesses, and private homes that constitute the town are arranged along the roads according to a strict hierarchy, in which proximity to the common denotes their rank in the town's social order. On the common itself are the town hall, the Grange, the Congregational church, and, if it has sufficient lineage, a general store. Farther out are the Elks' lodge, other Protestant churches, remaining businesses, and the Catholic church. At the periphery lie the town dump and mobile-home parks.

Linear towns, in contrast, are laid out along one main road. The center of a linear town is the midpoint between its two ends. Unlike the center of a radiant town, it is not a fixed point. It migrates up and down the main street in response to relative rates of growth and decay occurring at either end. Linear towns are less aesthetic than radiant ones, but they are more egalitarian. They are also easier for visitors, who can be sure that, simply by traveling from the

WELCOME TO ——— sign at one end to the YOU ARE NOW
LEAVING ———, COME AGAIN sign at the other, they have
seen everything, and if they didn't find a McDonald's or a
gas station, there isn't one.

Dumster is a linear town, strung out along Route 5 in a
north-south direction. It has one traffic light, located at the
junction of Main Street and Hill Street. The traffic light was
installed in 1954 by the Dumster Rotary, which thought it
would give the town a little radiance, something that Rotarians by nature are inclined to favor. In order to enhance the
effect of the light, they suggested that different names be
given to the two halves of Main Street created by this land-
mark. The Rotarians offered to sponsor a contest to pick
the names. The selectmen discussed the project. They liked
the idea, but they wondered about the cost of putting up
two street signs. Rotary agreed to pay for the signs too.

Jerry Bouchard won the contest. His winning entries were
North Main and South Main.

The light came with a button to stop traffic for pedestri-
ans. The button was installed on a lamppost in front of
Ernie's Barber Shop, which was about fifty feet from the
light. To put the button any closer would have involved
erecting another pole. This would have added considerably
to the cost of the project. Although the location was not very
convenient, it pleased the Bouchard family, since Jerry's
father, Ernest, was proprietor of the barber shop. Below the
button was a small plaque upon which was inscribed:

COURTESY OF DUMSTER ROTARY
IN MEMORY OF JERRY BOUCHARD
1954

Jerry was a little upset about the "In Memory" part since,
he said, that was what you wrote for dead people, but as the

Rotarians explained, they couldn't very well write "In Honor of," because it wasn't, and "Street Names by Jerry Bouchard" sounded like he was a fashion designer. So "In Memory" it was.

The plaque was more expensive than the Rotarians had anticipated, and they didn't have enough money left over to connect the button to the light. It didn't really matter. The only time it might have been used was at three o'clock, when shifts changed at Acme Tool and Die, and then there was always a policeman stationed at the intersection.

If one were to fly over Main Street (which as far as I know no one ever has, since it is not on the way anywhere, and there is no one in Dumster who owns a plane that he might fly over it in), it would look about the same at both ends. But when one drives into town, it is obvious that the two halves are not at all equal.

South Dumster is heavily influenced by those immigrants who came to Dumster to escape urban unemployment and eventually made their fortunes in rural underemployment. Hardworking people, they'd been attracted to Dumster by Acme Tool and Die, which in its heyday employed almost one thousand workers. At the entrance to South Dumster stands the Block, beckoning, like the Statue of Liberty, to the tired, the poor, and the huddled masses yearning to live cheap. And to the Snides.

The Snides are a collection of vaguely related individuals who own most of the businesses on South Main. In addition to the Block, which was their most recent acquisition (purchased from the umpteenth Flatlander who had sunk a small fortune into the building on the mistaken assumption that Dumster had an upper middle class waiting for the Block to be gentrified so they could move in), the Snides own Snide's Army-Navy, Snide's Mini Mart, Snide's Consignment, Snide's Laundromat, and Snide's Diner. All of the Snide businesses are but marginally profitable — profitable because of the Snide management philosophy, and marginally so for the same reason.

If someone were to write a book about the Snide theory of business management, it might be titled *More from Less,* and the subtitle would be, "No Product Too Poor to Sell. No Customer Too Poor to Buy." The first chapter of the book would describe, as exemplifying this philosophy, the Ritual of the Wet Straws.

Snide's Diner is located on the east side of South Main, about halfway between the light and the Block. The lot on which the diner sits is covered with gravel. The Snides picked gravel for their landscaping because it was cheap, required no maintenance, and was not conducive to hanging out. An unexpected benefit was aesthetic. Because the gravel matched the diner in color, it imparted to the building an impression, if not quite of majesty, at least of substantiality.

Snide's Diner is managed by Billy Snide. Billy is not very smart. Most of his customers are either old men with nothing better to do or young kids with many things better to do, who don't want to do them. Billy is smart enough to run Snide's Diner.

Inside the diner is a long counter. On the counter is a cylindrical glass straw holder, the kind that somebody designing an old-fashioned ice cream parlor would consider just the right thing to add a touch of authenticity to the place, but that Billy uses simply because it was there when he took over. The Ritual of the Wet Straws centers around the straw holder. When Billy isn't looking, one of the kids fills the holder with Coke. Upon discovery of this act of vandalism, Billy flies into a rage, fetches his broom, and shoos the kids out of the diner. Then he launches into the closest he ever comes to extended speech: a one-minute tirade on the evil nature of children who have nothing better to do than hang out — pronouncing *hang out* as a single word with the accent on the first syllable and using it interchangeably as verb or noun. During his monologue, Billy removes all the straws from the container, carefully places them on a cookie sheet, and puts them in the oven to dry. Having restored the straws to their original state of humidity, if not of color and texture, he returns them to the straw holder, which in the meantime he has emptied by pouring the Coke back into the soda machine. During summer vacation Billy's straws, like the kids, acquire a dark tan. The kids consider this great sport, and the old men think it good entertainment. All Billy knows is that it sells Coke.

Corporate headquarters for Snide Enterprises is the Talbot Building, a two-story brick edifice that covers most of the west side of South Main. It was built in 1847 by Elmer Talbot, the patriarch of Dumster's sole indigenously wealthy family. Old Mr. Talbot, who at that time was young Elmer, came to Dumster from Boston in 1840 with a modest inheritance and an uncanny way with investments. He used his inheritance to start a bank, and he used the bank to finance Acme Tool and Die Company, on the hunch — which even he did not fully understand — that Dumster seemed like a good place to start such a business. It turned out to be a pretty good hunch. Dumster had the perfect mix of people who could figure out how to design a machine to do a job and people who wanted to build those machines. Acme Tool and Die did so well that it spawned numerous offspring up and down the Connecticut River. From 1850 to 1970, the area was known as Machine Tool Valley. Dumster was its capital.

As Dumster prospered, so did Elmer. With the profits from Acme and a loan from his bank, Elmer built the first two-story business building in Vermont. It had retail stores at street level and offices on the second floor. On top of the building was a large block of marble. On it was engraved the single word *Talbot*. For the first hundred and twenty years it was the Talbots' frontispiece. For the last fifteen, it has been their headstone.

When Elmer died in 1885, he had amassed a considerable fortune, which, with minimal attention, should have allowed his descendants to live quite comfortably for many generations. The later Talbots, however, like many of the passively prosperous, had talents better suited to the demand side of business than to the supply. Nevertheless, it would have taken until well into the twenty-first century for their efforts to deplete the family financial reserves had they not been assisted considerably in their endeavors by the Japanese, who, by adding robotics to tool-and-die making, managed to render obsolete in one decade Dumster's one-hundred-and-twenty-year accumulation of machine tools, machine-tool makers, and machine-tool owners. In 1972 the family sold Acme Tool and Die to Consolidated Foods. Recognizing the great contribution Acme Tool and Die had made to Dumster, Consolidated retained the old name for their new business, only shortening it to Acme in order to avoid confusion about the factory's new function, which was assembling Japanese bicycles. The new plant had a work force about one-third that of Acme Tool and Die, and the wages it paid were in similar proportion.

The blight that had caused Acme Tool and Die to wither on the industrial vine spread rapidly to other Talbot businesses. The bank was left with a pile of foreclosed mortgages that were useless, since no one who could afford to buy them would have any reason to move to Dumster. The Talbot Building, sturdy enough to withstand anything except obsolescence, lost its tenants as stores on the ground floor auctioned off their accumulated inventory and inhabitants of the second floor moved to other towns where there were people who had money to spend on people who had offices. By 1974 the building resembled an abandoned fortress.

Within the species *Homo sapiens* there is a particular sub-species that, like its insect counterpart, thrives on that for which the rest of us no longer have any use. Taxonomically speaking, the Snides were members of this family, *Homo cockroachensis*. Nobody is sure where the Snides came from. All the town knows is that one day about twenty-five years ago, Clarence Snide, dressed in his faded gray suit, got off the bus in front of the post office with a large steamer trunk and a small satchel. He went straight to the Talbot Building, where he rented an office that to this day is still his . . . well, not really home, for that would be impossible . . . place of residence. The trunk was never seen again, but the satchel accompanied him wherever he went, as much a part of him as his dour stare. Every few weeks after that for the next year, the bus deposited another Snide on the sidewalk. By the end of that year the clan numbered about twenty, a population at which it stands today.

Since Clarence did not bring with him to Dumster any information on his background, the townspeople filled the void with the only material at their disposal. Rumors. The rumors hinted at ill-gotten means and unnatural breedings and were generally of the sort that, for ordinary business-men, would be disastrous to their enterprise. But for the Snides the rumors were salutary. They enhanced the im-pression that the Snides were possessed of special powers with respect to making money, and that if one did business with them, a little might rub off.

Clarence bought the Talbot Building from John Wilbur Talbot in 1975. The story goes that Clarence went into John Wilbur's office, put five thousand dollars down on the table, and said he wanted to buy the building. John Wilbur then said to Clarence did he think he was a fool or something to sell the building at that price, at which point Clarence fished into his pocket, took out a dollar bill, threw it on the table, and said, "Take it or leave it." And John Wilbur took it. It is a typical Snide story. Whether or not it is true does not matter. What matters is that it exists.

Clarence filled the stores on the ground floor with businesses, each one of which was run by a family member. Their success depended not only on the Snide name, but also on the fact that there was no competition. Unless one counted — which no one did — Contremond's General Store. Dan Contremond, its owner, was one of those uncommon people who folks like to believe is not: an honest man. Dan Contremond was also stubborn. He hung on to a business that lost money every year because he wouldn't change it, and for which, like the ton of cast-iron cookware he had in stock, there was no longer any market — except perhaps from tourists who were looking for a touch of Old Vermont to put in their new kitchen. But tourists didn't shop in Dumster.

Adjacent to the Talbot Building, on the corner of Hill and Main, is a fire-scarred building. The old Federal Building, a large wood structure, had housed the Federal District Court and the Dumster Post Office until 1965, when the former left town and the latter moved to a new home up the street. Clarence Snide bought the building in 1977. He planned to convert it into apartments. Everybody agreed that apartments were a smart thing to do with the building. Everybody, that is, except the state building inspector, who informed Clarence that in order to conform to the state housing code, the wiring would have to be replaced, and he would have to put fire escapes to the second floor. Shortly after Clarence got this news, the building caught fire at two o'clock in the morning. If the fire truck hadn't happened to be returning from a chimney fire and driven past the building just as the blaze started, it would have burned to the ground. The firemen managed to put out the fire, but not before the second floor collapsed. Miraculously, the roof remained intact, so that after the fire was put out the building looked much as it had before, only one story shorter. The townspeople all praised the fire department for doing such a good job. Even Clarence was impressed. "Shoulda burned to the ground," he said.

The cause of the fire was never exactly determined. The state fire marshal said it was "of suspicious origin." Clarence blamed it on the wiring. Nobody could understand why Clarence would pay for electricity in an unoccupied building. "For the alarms," Clarence said. He never bothered to explain what alarms. They certainly weren't fire, and there wasn't anything worth protecting from burglars. Clarence collected the insurance money, and that was the last he did with his investment. He didn't rebuild it, and he didn't tear it down. He just left it.

The selectmen declared the site to be a health hazard and a public nuisance. They issued an order telling Clarence to raze the building within ninety days. Clarence ignored the order. The selectmen consulted the town attorney. She said they could sue Clarence, and that they would probably win, but she couldn't promise anything, and she would need a retainer to look into it. The selectmen, after lengthy discussion, decided to table the matter, and so the ruins stand untouched, a fitting memorial to Dumster's war against the Snides.

6

There are no Snides on North Main. Lining both sides of the street are the great old homes of Dumster's past. Set back from the road behind white picket fences, immaculately groomed lawns and freshly painted houses testify to the civic pride of their owners. Between the street and the sidewalk are beautiful flowering crabs, maintained by the town as its one extravagance. On the east side of North Main, closer to the center of town, are Contremond's General Store, the First National Bank, and a small park. On the opposite side of the street are Smith's Top-Notch Hardware, the new post office, Old North Church, and a home for senior citizens that looks as if it might once have been a private home except that inside, it has so many tiny rooms and narrow stairways that you couldn't imagine any one family actually living there.

None did. It is the Old Dumster Hospital. When the Joint Commission on Accreditation of Hospitals finally discovered in 1976 that Dumster had a hospital and decided to make an inspection, it couldn't believe it was actually used to treat patients. After the inspection was finished, a total of one hundred and twenty-four violations had been found. JCAH told the town that if it wanted to keep its hospital, it would have to build a new one.

The people of Dumster liked having a hospital close to home, so they decided to build a new one. Several of the neighboring towns, which were no bigger than Dumster, had nice, new hospitals. The selectmen asked their neighbors where they got the money to build them. "Hill-Burton," the neighbors said.

The selectmen appointed Chester Davis to look into the matter. Chester found out that in 1946, Representative Lister Hill of Alabama and Senator Harold Burton of Ohio introduced a bill the purpose of which was

> to assist the several States to construct public and other non-profit hospitals for furnishing adequate hospital service to all the people.

The bill contained an appropriation of twenty-five million dollars, which Congress could give to small towns around America in order to help them build small hospitals. Back then hospitals were generally considered, like libraries and post offices, to be something every self-respecting town should have. Back then a day's stay in the hospital cost about twenty-five dollars.

The bill became a law. Everyone liked it. Voters who had never dreamed they would have the chance to stay in their own hospital liked it. Doctors and nurses and hospital administrators who wanted to live somewhere where they could plant tomatoes and chop down trees liked it. Contractors who lived in small towns loved it. All over the country little hospitals sprang up in little towns.

After Chester reported on Hill-Burton, the selectmen wrote a letter to Washington apologizing for not having been in touch sooner and asking if it could send some money, please, so that they could build a hospital and carry out the will of Congress.

Unfortunately they were a little late. Congressman Hill had died, Congressman Burton had retired, and hospitals cost about one hundred and fifty dollars a day. Congress had taken the economic pulse of the nation and found it to be weak. Hill-Burton was scrapped and replaced with PL 89–749. At first glance, PL 89–749 sounded just like Hill-Burton:

> The Congress declares that fulfillment of our national purpose depends on promoting and assuring the highest level of health attainable for every person. . . .

Later on, however, it turned out that this highest level of health

> depend[ed] on close intergovernmental collaboration and comprehensive planning at every level of government.

To which end Congress appropriated more money. This time, however, it was not for hospitals. It was for comprehensive health-planning agencies — one in every state except California, which had five. These agencies were empowered to review the medical needs of all the small towns in America to decide if they really needed their hospitals.

In order to help these agencies do their job, the government hired planners and experts and other kinds of serious-thinking people. People who needed offices. Since the purpose of the agencies was to save money, they couldn't very well go out and build new offices. Fortunately, they didn't have to. They just moved into the hospitals that had been vacated.

The population of Dumster in 1960 was three thousand, four hundred and twenty. By 1972 it had increased to three thousand, four hundred and sixty-four. Within twenty miles of Dumster there were three other hospitals, each one of which was about half full. The state health-planning agency considered the town's request. It did some studies, hired a few consultants, and made some projections. Then it wrote a report. The report said that, based on current use and projected demand, and taking into account certain other variables, Dumster would be eligible for a 3.6-bed hospital.

When the people of Dumster heard this, they said thank you very much, but a 3.6-bed hospital was not quite what they had in mind. The selectmen called a special town meeting to discuss the problem. "We want a hospital," said the people. "It's not in the budget," said the selectmen. "So what!" said the people. The selectmen talked it over. "To hell with the budget," they said, "the people have spoken." They authorized the town manager to build a sign.

The sign was placed at the intersection of Main and Hill. It was white and had a huge red thermometer painted on it. On top it said EMMELINE TALBOT MEMORIAL HOSPITAL FUND DRIVE. On the bottom it said IT'S UP TO US.

Emmeline Talbot was the name of Elmer Talbot's wife. The selectmen picked this name for the hospital in the hope that the Talbot family would be pleased and make a sizable contribution to the fund drive. Unfortunately, they forgot that the mother of Elmer's children was not Emmeline but Marion. Emmeline was Elmer's second wife, whom he married after Marion died at the age of thirty-eight. Emmeline was a very severe woman who felt that Marion had been lax in her control over the children. She bent all of her considerable will to correcting the mistake. The children called her Iron Finger because of her habit of poking them with her index finger whenever she wanted their attention. By the time the selectmen had realized their error, it was too late: the sign had already been painted.

Everyone pitched in. The hospital auxiliary had a bake sale. The American Legion sold flags in front of the bank. The Grange knitted placemats on which was embroidered *"It's Up to Us."* The fire department put on a chicken barbecue. Rotary held a penny sale. The Catholic church organized a three-day Bingothon. Businesses were asked to make donations for which they would get a hospital room named in their honor. Even Clarence Snide contributed. When the fund drive was all over, the red line just reached the top of the thermometer.

On July 4, 1973, Dumster celebrated Independence Day with the grand opening of Emmeline Talbot Memorial Hospital. It had twenty-two beds, an emergency room, an operating room, and doctors' offices. There was even a two-bed intensive-care unit in case somebody got really sick. The ICU was located in the northwest corner of the building, which bordered on Bill Easton's farm. Bill was partial to cows, but his wife had a broader scope of animal interests. On any given morning, a patient recovering from a heart attack might wake up and look out his window to find himself eye to eye with a llama, a pair of beefalos, or some Andalusian sheep. When the Accreditation Commission came back to inspect the new hospital, it said the animals would have to go. Mr. Shiftley asked what harm could there be in having people look at animals. Marius Bureaucratis, the head of the delegation, explained that patients recovering from a heart attack sometimes get disoriented. Seeing the llamas, they might forget where they were and think they were about to be trampled by a stampeding herd. They could have another heart attack. They could jump out of bed and break a leg. They could even think they were going crazy and become very depressed. Mr. Shiftley admitted that he hadn't thought of those possibilities. Dr. Bureaucratis said that was OK, it was his job to think of things like that.

Dr. Bureaucratis does his job well. There is a test given to elementary school children called "What Is Wrong with This Picture?" In the picture, there may be a table with one leg missing, or a door with no handle, or a cow with antlers. Students are asked to identify all the mistakes. The purpose of the test is to evaluate a student's powers of observation. There are twelve mistakes in the picture. Some students don't see anything wrong with the picture. When these students grow up, they become politicians. The average student finds nine. A few identify all of them. When Marius took the test, he found seventeen mistakes.

Mr. Shiftley said they would hate to board up the windows or move the hospital. Dr. Bureaucratis said he could understand and was not trying to make things difficult. His only interest was in protecting the patients. He thought about the situation and decided that if the patients signed a consent form saying they would not be frightened by the animals, then it would probably be all right, but he would check on it when he came back next time.

The people of Dumster were quite proud of their new hospital. They put a big sign on the front lawn. The sign said

EMMELINE TALBOT MEMORIAL HOSPITAL
IT WAS UP TO US

Before I came to Dumster, I thought a small hospital was one with less than three hundred beds. Emmeline Talbot seemed more like a doll hospital. But it worked. And it worked so well that, as I discovered, it did a far better job of treating those problems it could handle than the larger, fancier models. Not because it had a prettier view from its windows, or because of its doctors. Doctors in the hospital come and go, talking of diseases so, that they don't make much difference to patients. Emmeline Talbot was better because it was a nicer place to stay. It was nice to stay there because of the nurses.

Such as Sarah Trotter, the head nurse at Dumster Hospital. Sarah is a remarkable person. This is not surprising: most nurses are remarkable. They have to be.

------◄ ♦ ►------

SERIOUS READER NOTE: Nursing is a very demanding profession. To start with, nurses must learn everything a doctor learns, so that whenever a situation arises that might develop into a mistake on the part of the doctor if the nurse did what the doctor ordered instead of what he meant to do, the nurse can distinguish the latter from the former and prevent the mistake from occurring. Then nurses must learn how to use this knowledge so that neither the doctor nor the patient is aware they possess it, for in the former instance, it might cause the patient to lose confidence in the doctor, and in the latter, it might cause the doctor to lose confidence in himself. Finally, if, despite a nurse's best efforts, things are not going well between doctor and patient, and the nurse can't patch it up, the nurse must take the blame.

Nurses are very patient. They realize their reward will not be in this lifetime, for to receive even a fraction of the recognition they deserve would be to lessen the importance of the doctor. Nurses often believe in reincarnation.

------◄ ♦ ►------

If there were such a thing as an excellent nurse, which, for reasons that should be obvious by now, there isn't, Sarah would be one. She is very competent and very comforting. She almost makes you want to be sick, just so she can take care of you. Sarah is not very old, but is she not young either. She is neither fat nor thin. And she is not remarkably tall nor unduly short. She may be attractive, I am not sure.

I realize this is not a very helpful description, but I can't help it. Being a nurse, and especially wearing a nurse's uniform, creates a kind of shield around a person — one that can be penetrated by the eye so that you can see that there is a body there, but not by the other senses that are used to store in your brain the details of what a person's body is really like.

Sarah never gets upset. Whether dealing with an unreasonable patient or an unruly surgeon, she is always calm, and pleasant. This is very important, for unpleasantness has no place in our relationship — unpleasantness by Sarah, that is. A sensitive doctor needs someone like Sarah upon whom he can unburden his professional soul whenever he is overworked or underappreciated. Someone who, however similarly overworked and underappreciated she may be, knows better than to expect in return the sympathy she needs. Sarah had succumbed once to an excess of such sympathy and married a doctor. She parcels it out more carefully now.

For me, being with Sarah was like listening to Pachelbel's Canon in D, especially the beginning part that makes you feel like being with someone. Not necessarily doing anything. Just being. Sharing the illusion that you are sharing an illusion. However, I must admit (since this is a diary and I promised to be truthful) that under certain circumstances the feeling changes, such as when we are working together over a sick patient. Then, there occasionally springs up between us a peculiar kind of intimacy. (Sex fiends should not get too excited. Nothing is going to happen here.) The result of this intimacy is that I know more about the color of her nails and the shape of her knuckles than the color of her eyes or the shape of her lips. At times like that the tempo picks up and it feels more like the second part of the Canon, where you get a definite feeling that something is going to happen . . . except that nothing does, because the music ends first.

For the serious readers, who are probably wondering what's going on here, I should explain that my relationship with Sarah has no more to do with Pachelbel's Canon than it does with Romeo and Juliet.

When I finished the diary and sent it off to my agent, she told me it lacked security. I asked her what she meant.

"Most people aren't going to feel very secure when they find out they are going to be reading about Vermont," she said. "Unless, of course, you intend for only Vermonters to read your book."

I assured her that I didn't.

"Then the book needs something to reassure the reader who is afraid to wander too far into the literary forest. Something that makes him feel safe. Like his *New York Times.*"

I understood. I have seen the people from the city go to Contremond's on Sunday morning to get their *Times,* only to find that it is not there. They ask Dan what time he expects it. He says, "Don't." So they wait. When the papers finally arrive, Dan laboriously assembles them, interrupting his task at every possible opportunity to serve a customer, after which, returning to the papers, he says, "Now what was I doing? Oh, yes. The *Times.* Tricky paper, that *Times.* If it's as hard to read as it is to put together, must keep you busy pretty near all day." They get nervous. And Dan shuffles the sections around, wondering if they are all there, and assembles them so that no paper is complete until the last section — which is always Travel and Entertainment —

has been inserted in the middle. Then he counts the papers. "How many want a *Times*? Ten? Hmmm. Looks like I only got nine. Guess you'll have to share. Should be enough to go around. Or, I could auction them off. What'll it be, folks?" At which point the crowd starts to turn violent. "Wait a minute," Dan says. "Looks like I counted wrong. Here's an extra one stuck inside. Well, that's what happens when you rush a job."

It is for them that I mention Twining's and Pachelbel, so they can read on the jacket

> A passionate saga of life and death in the country, with an unforgettable cast of characters:
>
> · Doc, the outrageous but lovable, Twining's Earl Grey tea–drinking doctor
> · Sarah, the compassionate nurse, who makes Doc feel like Pachelbel's Canon in D

and feel that it would be OK to buy the book even if they never plan to read it.

Regardless of the type of music we made together, I enjoyed Sarah's company. It was my custom, upon arriving in the hospital, to visit the cafeteria first, in the hope that I might catch Sarah on her break and chat a bit before seeing patients.

Today was such a day. She was just sitting down to tea when I arrived.

"Hi, Sarah."

"Good morning, Dr. Conger."

(When I first came from California, I thought it was disrespectful for fellow professionals to address each other in this manner. I asked her to call me Beach. She refused. So I called her Nurse Trotter. She didn't answer.)

We reviewed the latest items of hospital gossip: an alleged affair between a doctor and a nurse — not good, she thought — and a rumor that the trustees would ban smoking in the cafeteria — well-intentioned but impractical. Then it was time to get down to business.

"Shall we go make rounds on the floor?" I asked.

"That would be fine."

———◆▸———

SERIOUS READER NOTE: Rounds on the floor is not a child's game. It is an ancient ritual of medicine, the purpose of which is to allow nurses to make sure that patients do not make doctors feel poorly. This can be difficult, because, as sensitive people, we are very susceptible to not feeling well. This is especially true when we are criticized.

Patients never fully appreciate just how sensitive doctors are. This is because patients get so wrapped up in their own problems that they don't think about how their behavior might affect the doctor. As a consequence, patients often do or say things that, although not intended to be critical, might be perceived as such by a sensitive person. This inconsiderate attitude on the part of patients is usually excused on the grounds that they are sick.

———◆▸———

The first patient we saw was Martin Fullum. Mr. Fullum had pneumonia. I had ordered penicillin for him. Ordinarily this would be a wise therapeutic step. However, when Mr. Fullum was a child, he got penicillin for a sore throat and almost died. He didn't tell me about this incident, perhaps because he was too embarrassed, or perhaps because I didn't ask him. When Sarah asked him if he was allergic to penicillin, he said yes.

Before we got to the bedside, Sarah brought me Mr. Fullum's chart. "I'm very sorry, Dr. Conger, but I haven't done your orders yet. You ordered something that looks like penicillin, but I know it can't be since he is allergic to penicillin. Was it panamycin you wanted him to have?"

"Yes, Sarah, it was."

"Thank you very much. That's what I thought."

The next patient was an older man who had fallen down the cellar stairs after making a wrong turn on his way to the bathroom. He had come into the emergency department with his scalp split open, and it had taken several hours for me to put him back together. I started to unwrap his dressing to see how my needlepoint was faring. Sarah tapped me gently on the shoulder. "Did you want me to get your sterile gloves before or after you washed your hands, Dr. Conger?"

The last patient was Abigail Carter. Abigail had a bad case of arthritis in her knees. I had done everything I could think of to alleviate her symptoms. I prescribed pills. I gave her injections. I took X rays. I sent her to physical therapy. I consulted an orthopedic surgeon. I even talked with her. A normal patient exposed to this therapeutic barrage would at least make some effort to hobble around so that I could see my efforts weren't wasted. Not Abigail. When I asked her how she was doing, she said if this was the best I could do, I might as well cut her legs off and be done with it.

After we had finished with her, Sarah said, "Mrs. Carter has been very difficult. She won't do her exercises, and she refused her medicine this morning. I'm afraid she doesn't have a very positive attitude toward her illness. It's a shame she can't see how much better she is. I think it's just wonderful, all that you've done for her."

"You're right, Sarah. Maybe I should get a psychiatric consultation with Dr. Shrank."

"Oh, that's an excellent idea. Patients always seem to stop complaining after they have a talk with him."

We went back to the nurses' station. While I was making my notes, the medical records clerk came up to me and asked please, would I sign the chart that had been sitting on my desk for two months, because otherwise the hospital wouldn't get paid for the patient's stay. It was just the kind of straw that breaks a busy doctor's back. I threw the chart across the room, jammed my pen into the telephone receiver, and stomped down the corridor.

Sarah caught up with me in the hall, put her arm around my shoulder, and guided me to the cafeteria, where she fetched me a cup of tea. Then she sat down.

"Oh, Dr. Conger," she said, "you're working too hard. I wish you'd take some time off. Just for yourself. You've earned it."

I am very grateful to Sarah, and I try to show it whenever I can. But, as a sensitive person, it is difficult for me to praise her in public or defend her when patients blame her for mistakes I have made. However, every Valentine's Day I give her and all the other nurses a big box of chocolates . . . so they will know how much I appreciate them.

7

My science teacher in high school was named Peter Tock. We called him Mr. Z. He thought the Z stood for Zorro, and considered the nickname a sign of affection.

Mr. Tock had a very large nose. On the end of his nose was a giant pimple. His nickname came from the pimple. We called it Old Faithless. Old Faithless had been on Mr. Z's nose for almost twenty years without ever erupting. To those of us in the prime of our acne careers, Old Faithless evoked both fascination and horror: fascination because we couldn't believe a pimple could get so large without popping; and horror because its presence on the face of an old man was a portent of what might happen to us did we not properly attend to our own disfigurements.

The reason the pimple never erupted was because it wasn't a pimple at all. It was a basal cell epithelioma. A skin cancer. And all the time Mr. Z was waiting for it to pop and be done with, it was actually burrowing in deeper and deeper, like the taproot of a dandelion. Finally one day a colleague (there was no Mrs. Tock, else the pimple would have disappeared long ago) said to him, "Don't you think you ought to have that looked at?," and the doctor had to carve off most of his nose to save his face.

Mr. Z's favorite subject was weights and measures. He felt that our ability to divide any large and indeterminate substance into small, identical parts was proof of a very important principle. He never explained exactly what the principle was, but he implied it might have to do with God.

"History may seem pretty complicated," he said, "but when you think about the fact that the Roman Empire consisted of exactly thirty-one billion, five hundred and thirty-six million seconds, which is only thirty-one million times the number of seconds you took to eat breakfast, it all falls into place."

Mr. Z's theory had a ring of fairness to it. Everything was the same, only in slightly different quantities. But it was dead wrong. Five hundred pounds of oil is worth a lot more than its equivalent weight in uncut, unsplit wood. The six hundred and fifty thousand seconds I have spent making my bed are worth nothing at all. And Monday morning means more than the entire rest of the week.

Especially the Monday morning after a weekend on call.

After three months in Dumster, I was still adjusting to general practice. In California, my job consisted of listening to my patients' complaints, considering the diagnostic possibilities, and then referring them to the appropriate specialist. I was a traffic cop, directing the flow of patients along medical highways, guaranteeing that each specialist got his share of business. It was not very demanding, but it was important work. Without it, the profession would degenerate into internecine warfare as orthopedists battled with neurosurgeons over bad backs, and gastroenterologists sparred with the surgeons for the rights to a peptic ulcer.

Dumster was not like California. My first patient on Saturday morning was George Bugbee. One of his cows had fallen on him while he was milking. He came in with a badly swollen ankle and toes that were pointing in the general direction of Boston. I knew that country doctors were expected to take care of problems like this, so I took the bull by the horns: I ordered an X ray. The X ray showed a fracture of the lateral malleolus with widening of the mortise, indicating disruption of the deltoid ligament. (I didn't know all this at the time. All I knew was that the black spaces and the white spaces didn't match up the way they were supposed to. I showed the films later to Fred Cracker, our orthopedic surgeon. He told me what it was.)

"You've got a broken ankle," I told Mr. Bugbee.

"I know."

"You need an orthopedic surgeon."

"I need a cast."

"It's displaced," I explained. "I've never reduced a fracture before." I thought that explanation was enough to justify referring him.

"I never broke my ankle before," he replied, indicating he was willing to take a chance with me.

So, with Ella Maxham, the emergency-room nurse, supervising and George assisting, I reduced the fracture and wrapped the ankle in enough plaster to withstand mortar fire.

"Not a bad job, Doc," said George as he struggled to lift his leg. "Won't have to worry about blowing away in a storm."

"When he comes back, you take it off," Ella said.

The whole weekend was like that. One after another they came in. Lacerations from chain saws, dislocated shoulders, metal chips in the eye. Ella would guide me patiently through each case and afterward tell me what a good job I had done. By Monday morning I was tired. A sensitive person who is tired is particularly susceptible to setbacks. I needed a good Monday morning.

I walked into my office. Sitting on my desk was a fresh pot of tea and two of Maggie's homemade blueberry muffins.

They were still warm. I looked at my appointment book. First on the list was William Fusswood.

Normal patients come to see me because they have a particular problem. They tell me about it, listen to my advice, and then they leave. Sometimes they tarry, not because they especially value my opinion, but because it makes us both feel better to chat a bit.

Most people do not relish their opportunities to play the part of patient, and when asked to do so, their performance is indifferent. Not Fusswood. Time after time, when the curtain goes up, he plays his role with a gusto that makes all other actors look like little more than walk-ons. Even the doctor.

To emerge from an encounter with Fusswood and retain enough energy to keep doctoring for the rest of the day requires, as Maggie wisely knew, prior sustenance.

Fortified by my tea, I walked into the examining room. Fusswood was sitting in the chair.

If he hadn't been the only person sitting in a very small room, I might not have noticed him at all. He was a slightly built man: slightly overweight, slightly balding, and slightly disheveled. William Fusswood resembled a pair of pants that had been worn one day too long and would look better if they were pressed, but would probably be OK if nobody looked at them too closely. Which nobody was likely to do, for Fusswood looked just like the millions of other middle-aged men who unobtrusively dot the American landscape. His only distinguishing feature was his posture. When he walked, he did not face straight ahead but at an angle, so that as he moved, he appeared to be struggling to maintain his direction, as if his body were a shopping cart that had one defective wheel, and you had to work it pretty hard to keep it going where you wanted it to.

Fusswood didn't wait for me to ask how he was.

"I was watching the news last night, and I got a sharp

pain. Right over my heart." He pointed to an area below his left nipple where no self-respecting heart would be caught dead. "And last week my brother in Newark had a heart attack. He's only thirty-seven. Two years younger than me. I'm scared."

"A natural feeling, Fusswood. But there's no need to worry. Your pain does not sound cardiac in origin. And I suspect your brother's trouble comes from the stress of city living. You're safe out here in the country."

"He don't live in the city, Doc. He lives in Newark, Vermont. Up in the Northeast Kingdom. The biggest city he's ever been to is St. Johnsbury."

"I see. In that case, we may have to start you on a risk-modification program."

"What's that?"

"Risk modification involves changing your life-style to give you new, healthy habits in place of your old, unhealthy ones. Like smoking. Smoking is very bad for the heart."

"That's what Doc Franklin said. But I can't stop now. It's too late."

"It's never too late to improve your health."

"It is when you quit last New Year's."

"That was not a wise decision, Fusswood. Premature termination of unhealthy habits is generally not a good idea. It leaves a person with nothing to do when his health is really on the line. Fortunately, there are plenty of eggs in the risk-modification basket. I suggest we start with reducing your cholesterol level. It's quite popular these days."

"Listen, Doc. I haven't seen the inside of an egg in two weeks. All I put on my toast now is carrot scrapings. I ran five miles yesterday. I threw away my salt shaker. And I enrolled in a yoga course."

Fusswood was on a disease-prevention orgy. I was going to have to try a different approach to settle him down.

"That's an impressive set of accomplishments. You must

73

be doing wonders for your coronaries. With habits like those, your risk of getting a heart attack in the next year is practically nil. In fact, I would say you are just about invincible."

"That's what they said about the *Titanic*. Pretty good isn't good enough. I gotta know for sure. I need a stress test."

I should have seen it coming. Every middle-aged man who gets a twitch between his nose and his navel wants to prove his immortality with a stress test.

"Take off your shirt and get on the table." I placed my stethoscope on his chest and listened for a few seconds. Then I frowned.

"How good is your life insurance policy?"

Fusswood paled. "What do you mean? Don't beat around the bush, Doc. Give it to me straight."

"You have myocardius ossificans. Stone heart. I expect you will die within the week."

He gasped, looked at me hard for a few seconds, and then grinned. "You're putting me on."

"Congratulations, Fusswood. You passed your stress test."

"I don't mean that kind of stress test," he protested. "I mean the one where you hook me up to the wires and watch my heart on TV while I run."

"An exercise electrocardiogram. I'll order one, if you insist. But it could be a dangerous proposition."

"I've heard it's no problem in the proper hands. But, if you can't do it . . ." He shrugged and started to put on his shirt.

"The test itself is quite safe. It is the results I am concerned about."

"Whatta you mean?"

"You feel pretty good right now, don't you?"

"Sure. But I don't want anything to happen to my ticker. Replacement parts are hard to get."

"Suppose you fail the test?"

"How could I? You just said yourself that I look great. I feel great. I can beat any machine." Tentatively, he suggested, "You're joking again."

"I'm afraid not. I've had patients in better shape than you fail their exercise test."

Fusswood gulped. "Well, I guess I'd ... Why, I'd do whatever you told me to do. That's what I came here for."

"Suppose I told you to stop running?"

"Why would tell me to do that?"

"Think about it. You come in for a checkup. I tell you your heart is a little weak, but it's no big deal, and you can keep on running. Then one day you drop dead while running down the street. How does that make me look?"

"Could that really happen?"

"Sure could. People with heart disease are about four times more likely to die during exercise than at rest."

"I guess I'll have to take up knitting." Fusswood managed a weak smile.

"It's not that easy. People in lousy shape are much more likely to get heart attacks than those who are fit."

"So you're telling me that if I got a bad heart, it's dangerous to exercise and it's dangerous not to exercise?"

"Exactly."

"That doesn't make sense."

"I don't make the facts, Fusswood. I just report them."

"Yeah. Well, listen. I'm not paying this kind of money for you to be a reporter. There must be something you can do for me."

"There is. Take the test. If you fail, I'll call you a false positive."

"You saying I'm a phoney?" Fusswood said angrily.

"Not you, Fusswood. The test. It says you have a problem, when you really don't. The test lies."

"Why would it do that?"

"Beats me. A lot of tests are like that. Highly untrustworthy. But don't worry about it. There's a way to tell if the test is wrong. I can send you up to Hanover to have an arteriogram."

"What's an arteriogram?"

"They stick a catheter into your heart and squirt dye into your arteries to see what kind of shape they're in. If the arteriogram shows any are plugged, you get a coronary-artery-bypass graft. They take a vein from your leg and use it to make detours around those vessels that are blocked."

"How can they do that while the heart is pumping?"

"They don't. When they do a bypass they stop the heart. But don't worry. They can usually start it up again without any trouble. In fact, your chances of survival are better than ninety-five percent."

"All this because of a few squiggles on the EKG machine?"

"That's the price you pay for violating the first law of testing: never order a test upon the results of which you are not prepared to act."

"What the hell does that mean?"

"If I suspect that you have a particular condition, and I order a test to find out, the test must be damn good at telling whether or not you have that condition; and, before I order the test, we must have a treatment plan which you agree to follow if I find trouble. I told you the risk of dying from a heart attack was higher with exercise. That's true, but it's a relative risk. Since you don't spend most of your time running, what you really want to know is the absolute risk. For every million hours spent jogging by men over the age of forty, three will die. That figures out to about thirty-eight years of jogging for each death.

"How good is the stress test? If a person looks healthy when he takes the test, and he fails, the chances are two out of three that the test is wrong."

"If the test is no good, how come doctors do it?"

I waved my hands to indicate it was just one of those things.

"So you're telling me I should just turn around and walk out of here, pretend that I am in perfect health, and do whatever I please, even though I could drop dead at any minute?"

"Life's a gamble, Fuss."

"I don't buy it. I'll tell you what I need, and it ain't philosophy of life. I need a pill. And don't tell me about no goddam one aspirin a day keeping the doctor away. I want a real pill."

"Of course you do. Medical research is working hard to come up with something, and any day now, we should be getting a breakthrough."

"How about this cholewhatsitmean? I read in the newspaper that it cuts your risk of heart attacks in half."

I started involuntarily. The only thing I knew about cholestyramine, which I assumed was the drug in question, was that it was good for diarrhea. Fusswood obviously had additional information on the drug. It was an awkward situation. To admit ignorance would destroy Fusswood's confidence in me; on the other hand, to prescribe the drug simply on his hearsay could be equally embarrassing if his information turned out to be incorrect.

I am a conscientious doctor. I read my medical journals faithfully. And I go to seminars in Acapulco and Aspen every year to keep up on the latest developments. But I am a busy man, and I don't have the time to go poring through the newspaper every day to find out that some overly ambitious scientist has leaked classified medical information to an unscrupulous reporter, who — before the profession can thoroughly analyze and digest it — hands it over to the public just so patients can come in and embarrass their doctors. In the short run this may make them feel pretty smug, but when the chips are down and they need to have unquestioning faith in their doctors, and it isn't there, they will be very sorry indeed.

"Cholestyramine is a possibility. I have considered it in your case, and I was just about to mention it when you brought it up yourself. But it has many side effects. We will have to run some tests to see if it might help you. I will make an appointment for you to come back after I have the results, and we can make a decision at that time."

"Now you're talking."

I sent Fusswood off to the laboratory for some random blood work. Then I headed straight for the library.

When Fusswood returned the following week, I was ready for him.

"Well, Doc, how did I check out?"

"As I feared, Fusswood, the tests showed that cholestyramine is out of the question. Of course, if you would like to get another opinion . . ."

"That's OK, Doc. I trust you. I figured I was too far gone to help."

"On the contrary. You are quite healthy. That is precisely the problem."

"I don't understand. Are you saying I'm too healthy to take medicine to keep me from getting sick?"

"Exactly. Unless, of course, you want to take the pill to prevent somebody else's heart attack."

Fusswood was silent. He appeared to be reconsidering his refusal of my second-opinion offer. I proceeded with my exposition.

"It's all in the numbers. Cholestyramine reduces heart attacks by fifty percent. That sounds great on paper, but what does it mean? Two out of every thousand men like you are scheduled for a heart attack this year. One half of two is one. That means that nine hundred and ninety-nine of you must take cholestyramine in order to help that one lucky fellow. Considering the risks, that's quite a sacrifice."

"Risks?"

"Sixty of you will have to stop because of upset stomach, constipation, and malnutrition."

"That's not very appetizing, Doc. Isn't there anything else I could try that wouldn't be quite so risky?"

"There is. It's called placebo. Placebo is the standard against which all new drugs are tested. Over the years it's been used to treat many diseases. Usually it works as well as the drug it's being tested against. Sometimes better. They used it in the cholestyramine study. It worked about half as well as cholestyramine. The nicest thing about placebo is that it has absolutely no side effects."

"I'll take it, Doc. Script it on me."

"I afraid I can't."

"Why not?"

"Despite its excellent track record, the FDA has never approved placebo. Of course, I might be able to get some for you on the QT." I winked conspiratorially at him.

"No, thanks. I don't want to buck Uncle Sam. You sure there's no way I could make this cholestyramine work better?"

"Well. Yes, but it would mean some major changes in your life."

"Nothing's too major if it's good for the old ticker." Fusswood tapped his chest. "I'll do whatever you say."

"Stop running. Take up a more sedentary sport, like professional-football watching. Start smoking again — two packs a day at least. Finally, get rid of your granola. It's a three-eggs-and-bacon breakfast for you from now on."

Fusswood was confused. "But you just said — "

"That it would increase your risk of having a heart attack to do these things. Precisely the point. As your risk goes up, so does your benefit from cholestyramine. If, instead of the two-out-of-a-thousand bracket, you move into the two out of a hundred, we can get your odds of having a heart attack in the next ten years up to twenty-five percent. That means you've got better than a one-in-ten chance of being the lucky fellow who doesn't get a heart attack because he took cholestyramine."

Fusswood was not persuaded. "Thanks for trying, Doc, but I think I'll pass on cholestyramine."

"Then you have one option left, the only risk factor you haven't yet addressed: your family history. Right now the biggest threat to your health is your brother. Disown him, and your worries are over."

Fusswood smiled. "No problem, Doc. My wife never liked his kids anyway."

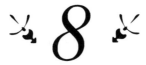

8

*F*usswood was not always a patient. He used to be just an ordinary person, no more inclined to go to a doctor for every somatic twitch or rattle than he would be to consult a mechanic whenever his gas gauge was low.

During my first week in Dumster, Fusswood came in for a checkup. It was not his idea. He was under direct orders from his wife, who wanted a professional review of her marital portfolio. I took his history. I examined him. I did some tests. Then we sat down to go over the results.

"Generally, you are in pretty good shape, Mr. Fusswood. There is, however, one slight abnormality which will require further evaluation. You have blood in your urine."

"You must be mistaken," he replied. "I've never seen any blood."

"This isn't blood you can see. It was found on microscopic examination."

"If it's that little, it hardly seems worth worrying about."

"It's not the amount that's important. It's what's causing it."

"Which is what?"

"I can't tell without further tests."

"I appreciate your interest, Doc. But I feel pretty good

right now, so I think I'll skip the tests. If I have any trouble with my waterworks, I'll get in touch."

I could tell there was no point in lecturing him on the value of early disease detection.

"It's your body. If you change your mind, let me know."

An hour after he left, his wife called to ask about the results of the examination. I told her about the blood in the urine and advised an X ray of the kidney.

On the X ray there was a peculiar shadow in the right kidney. The radiologist thought it was probably just a cyst, but couldn't be sure. But there was something peculiar about the left kidney. He recommended a CT scan.

The CT scan showed the right kidney was OK, but on top of the left was a lump. Kidney lumps were out of my department. I consulted our urologist, Dr. Elizabeth Flushing.

SERIOUS READER NOTE: If there are any male readers who feel squeamish about being examined by a woman doctor, you should not. There is no such thing as a woman doctor. I don't mean this in a biological sense; I mean in the functional, everyday sense. In the process of transforming students into doctors, all traces of their former existence are carefully removed. This is not so much to prevent their personal attributes from interfering with their treatment of patients as it is to prevent patients from confusing their doctors with ordinary human beings.

Dr. Flushing didn't know what the lump was. She thought it might be a good idea to look into the bladder. Looking into the bladder wasn't likely to tell much about the kidney, but she recommended it anyway because all doctors have their favorite thing to do when they don't know what is going on, and this was hers.

The bladder was normal. Dr. Flushing consulted a specialist in Boston. He advised injecting dye into the blood vessels to get a better picture of this lump.

Fusswood was admitted to the hospital for an angiogram. It determined that the lump was not part of the kidney.

Attention shifted from the kidney to the adrenal gland, which lives on top of the kidney and makes hormones. A urine test detected elevated levels of a hormone. I consulted an endocrinologist. He suggested blood tests. They were all normal.

By this time subtle changes began to appear in Mr. Fusswood's behavior. Initially he was completely indifferent to our flurry of diagnostic activity, convinced as he was that his health was perfect. Gradually, however, he began to take an interest in the problem.

He started asking me about the results of his tests, and he took a daily body inventory, hoping that he could find something that might be helpful in making the diagnosis.

"My fingernails have been kind of brittle the past few months. And when I eat pickles my tongue tingles. Do you think there might be any connection to the lump?"

"Quite possibly," I replied. I called for a dermatologist and an otolaryngologist, both of whom failed to shed any light on the matter.

I reviewed the case with my colleagues. They were of divided opinion as to etiology, but unanimous regarding treatment.

I discussed the situation with Mr. Fusswood.

"Can't you take it out?" he asked.

"Our sentiments exactly."

At surgery, the surgeons found a mass the size of a grapefruit. It was so large that they had to make an incision from his spine to his belly button in order to get it out. On pathological examination it turned out to be an unusually large collection of fat. We all agreed that it was a most unusual case. Even the specialist from Boston.

I broke the good news to Fusswood. He was not impressed.

"You mean I went through all this rigmarole just to get rid of a hunk of fat?" he said.

Fusswood had never been sick before. He was used to being in charge of his life and having his own opinion about things. Fusswood didn't know yet how a patient was supposed to respond in a situation like this.

Fortunately he was in the hospital, which was the perfect place to teach him. Especially if there is an operation involved.

SERIOUS READER NOTE: A hospital day is not constrained by those arbitrary boundaries that define an outside-world day: work and rest, light and dark, wake and sleep. A hospital day is a continuous life experience, like a train that travels on its circular track and stops from time to time at various stations along the way.

TWO A.M.: Fusswood is lying in his bed, trying to ignore the symphonic performance that is coming from the neighboring bed, in which resides a very sick patient. The ebb and flow of this patient's bodily functions are being monitored by numerous electronic devices connected to him by a maze of tubes and wires. The devices emit an assortment of melodic beeps and pings on a regular basis. There are also lower-pitched tones that seem to come from the patient, but they bear no resemblance to emanations from any of the body orifices with which Fusswood is familiar. Each time he starts to drift off to sleep, a new movement begins, and he awakens abruptly, wondering whether it is part of the intended orchestration, or a variation on the theme that should be called to the conductor's attention.

In comes a nurse, fresh-smelling and full of pep. She shines a flashlight in Fusswood's face.

"Are you asleep, Mr. Fusswood?"

Fusswood, hoping she will go away, does not answer. The nurse repeats her question. Fusswood grunts. Thus encouraged, she attempts to engage him in conversation. Fusswood does not respond. She offers him a sleeping pill.

"Sleep is very important in the healing process," she explains. "And it's not always easy to sleep in a hospital."

Fusswood gratefully accepts the offer.

Four A.M.: Fusswood is asleep. The nurse reappears. She has just had her lunch. Seafood salad, french fries, and apple pie. It was quite good, she tells him. Fusswood's lower lip begins to twitch.

"Your mouth seems awfully dry, Mr. Fusswood. Would you care for a throat swab?"

For the last two days Fusswood has dined exclusively on these culinary delights: cotton-tipped applicators containing an exquisite blend of machine oil and antiseptic, which are sure to tingle even the most discriminating of taste buds. This time, however, Fusswood declines.

"Time to check your vital signs again," she intones cheerfully. "We need to make sure you're still alive."

Fusswood says he believes such to be the case and asks if they could be dispensed with.

"Oh, no! I need them for morning report," implying that

such an omission could have dire consequences for his recovery. She checks his pulse, his blood pressure, and his temperature. Then she offers another sleeping pill. Although it is almost daylight, Fusswood has learned that nurses consider refusal of an offered pill to be a personal insult. He takes the pill.

After passing the time of night a bit, the nurse leaves to continue on her rounds, making sure that all her charges will be presentable for the next shift.

Fusswood settles into a deep sleep, which could, if uninterrupted, continue until the following evening.

During this sleep he dreams that he is on a sailboat in the middle of the ocean. It is nighttime. He is lying on the deck and looking at the sky. The stars are twinkling, and the sea is as smooth as glass. Waves lap against the side of the boat, rocking it gently to and fro. All is peaceful. Suddenly, a bolt of lightning flashes in the sky. It strikes the boat. Fusswood is thrown overboard. He swims toward the boat and tries to climb aboard. Something grabs him and pulls him back into the sea. It is an enormous octopus. Vainly he struggles to escape. His end seems imminent.

The octopus speaks.

"Seventy-nine point two."

Fusswood opens his eyes. The octopus is dressed entirely in white. "Don't be alarmed," says the octopus. "That's not your real weight. It's your weight in kilograms. Kilograms are part of the metric system. We're doing everything metric now. It's very scientific. Your real weight is one hundred and seventy-four pounds. Just in case you're interested."

Fusswood is not particularly interested. He is trying to figure out where his boat has gone. He thinks about asking the octopus but, never having talked to one before, is not sure how to address it. Wisely, he says nothing.

Gently the octopus places Fusswood back on his boat, and he immediately falls asleep.

SERIOUS READER NOTE: *Many patients are quite upset about being weighed in the middle of the night. I once had one who complained so, I wrote in his orders "Weigh patient at 9 A.M. daily." I considered the matter settled and thought no more of it.*

Until the next morning, when the patient, having been weighed at the usual time, angrily accused me of ignoring his request. I confronted Sarah with this flagrant flouting of my authority.

"I don't think you ever wrote the order," she said. "You were probably busy."

I insisted that I quite distinctly remembered writing the order. She suggested we look at the chart. To my surprise, she was right. No such order existed. Although I said nothing, traces of my suspicion must have shown on my face. Sarah became quite indignant.

"Beach!" she exclaimed, using my first name to emphasize I had strayed beyond the bounds of acceptable doctor-to-nurse behavior. "Nobody would disregard your orders. And nobody would tamper with a hospital record. You have too many important things to do to be worrying about daily weights. And you look awfully tired. I think what you need is a cup of tea."

At tea, I asked Sarah why it was necessary to weigh patients at such an ungodly hour. As always, Sarah had the answer.

"It is very important that a patient's weight be standardized to a particular time of day. This avoids the problem of fluctuations."

I wondered why his weight couldn't be standardized to a more respectable hour, but I could tell by the look on Sarah's face that my daily-weight lesson was over, and further questions would not be likely to provide additional enlightenment.

On the way back to the floor, Sarah explained how busy it was at nine o'clock, what with doctors making rounds and writing orders, and that it was important for the nurses be available to the doctors, and that things were much less hectic in the middle of the night. It was a very friendly chat, and Sarah made me feel, as always, that my slightest wish was her command. But I never wrote an order about daily weights after that.

Seven A.M.: Fusswood was greeted by another cheerful nurse, eager to brief him on his schedule of events for the day, which featured a visit to X ray and a chat with someone from the billing department.

Fusswood had trouble concentrating on the subject at hand. He was distracted by the object the nurse had set on his bedside table. It was a food tray — the first he had seen since his operation. In order to prevent Fusswood from getting too stimulated by the gastronomic treats that lay therein, the contents of the tray were discreetly concealed under metal covers.

"Enjoy your breakfast," said the nurse before he left.

Fusswood turned his attention to the tray. A card declared that the arrangement before him was BREAKFAST. In small print below, he was further informed that this particular BREAKFAST was something called *Full Liquids.*

Full Liquids sounded pretty exciting after two days of throat swabs, and Fusswood attacked the tray with gusto. To his disappointment, whatever the liquids were full of, it was not taste. This, it turned out, was provided separately in four identical paper packets, each bearing a tiny label, which, without his glasses, Fusswood could not read. But this didn't really matter, for in his drugged state, Fusswood did not possess the hand-eye coordination necessary to transfer the contents from one to the other.

Coffee. That would straighten him out. Finding a warm brown liquid in one of the containers, he took a gulp and waited for the lift that invariably accompanied his morning hit of caffeine.

Nothing happened. He took another gulp. Nothing. Fusswood was still waiting when the nurse returned.

"I see you're drinking your bouillon," he exclaimed encouragingly. "That's very good. Bouillon is high in protein. Now, finish it up like a good dear." He held the cup to Fusswood's lips.

Fusswood pushed it away. "Whersh coffee?" he asked belligerently.

"Coffee is out of the question, Mr. Fusswood," the nurse replied. "It contains caffeine. Caffeine is a drug. We wouldn't want to fill you full of drugs when you're trying to recover from an operation, would we?"

Eight A.M.: Fusswood was awakened abruptly by his incision, which informed him in no uncertain terms that it was not pleased. It wanted some attention, and it wanted it pronto. Fusswood rang the bell. His nurse appeared promptly.

"Hursh," Fusswood said, pointing to the incision.

The nurse inspected the wound. "It looks fine."

"Hurrshts!" Fusswood persisted. "Need shot!"

The nurse looked at him. Unshaven, unkempt, and almost unintelligible, Fusswood resembled more an applicant to the detox program than a postoperative patient.

"Stand up, please."

Fusswood got out of bed and rose slowly to his feet. Swaying unsteadily, he grabbed the nearest object for support. It was the tray table. This was an unfortunate choice. Fusswood tottered for an instant as the tray table slid gracefully away and then collapsed on the floor.

The nurse helped him back into bed. "Would you say Methodist Episcopal for me, Mr. Fusswood?" he asked once Fusswood was safely behind bars. "If you don't mind, that is," he added almost as an afterthought.

89

Why the nurse wanted to enter into a religious discussion with him at this time escaped Fusswood, but he was not about to question him. He wanted that shot.

"Missodish episotable," he replied in what seemed to him a pretty good approximation of his request.

It was not good enough.

"I'm sorry, Mr. Fusswood. I'm afraid you're still under the influence of the sleeping pills you got last night. It would be contraindicated to give you a pain shot now."

Fusswood said he would be willing to take this chance, but the nurse was adamant. Terrified by the prospect of being left alone with his angry incision, Fusswood racked his besotted brain for something that would make the nurse relent. Suddenly it came to him.

"Ashprin!"

"Dr. Conger hasn't ordered aspirin for your pain. Only morphine."

"Ashprin home," he protested. "Don't ask Conger."

"You are not at home now. You are in the hospital. Why don't you take a little nap, and I'll check you again in two hours." The nurse smiled again and left.

Noon: Fusswood finally got a shot at eleven o'clock, just in time to ruin his appetite for lunch. The nurse informed him that if he didn't do better with supper, he might have to put a feeding tube into his stomach. Otherwise he might not get enough nourishment for the wound to heal. He also told Fusswood that with a tube, there was a chance of pneumonia. Fusswood promised to do better next time. "That's the spirit," said the nurse and told him it was time for his trip to X ray.

The excursion to X ray was a welcome diversion. Fusswood had been staring at the ceiling in his room for the past three days and was eager to get out. While being wheeled through the corridors, he thought about the importance of ceilings to patients, and how nice it would be if they, like the walls, were decorated with paintings by local artists, so that he could appreciate them better.

Three P.M.: The man from the billing department was very friendly. He told Fusswood that his insurance policy, except for the incidentals, the deductibles, and the copayment, should cover most of the cost of his stay. Fusswood asked how much this meant he would have to pay. The man told him not to worry, they would be able to work things out once he got better.

Five P.M.: When supper arrived, Fusswood, still thinking about his discussion with the billing clerk, couldn't eat anything. He knew he would be in trouble if his failure was discovered, so he tried to disguise it by shuffling things around on his tray. The nurse was not fooled. She gave him a stern lecture on the importance of good nutrition and mentioned the possibility of a tube. Then she asked how he was feeling.

Fusswood by now was quite good at his state-of-the-body report. While in X ray, he had noticed rising up from the vicinity of his abdomen a rather large mound. Poking gingerly at the mound, he found it to be firm but not especially painful. Fusswood was quite worried about this development but had been afraid to mention it until asked for fear of getting known as an alarmist. Alarmists, he had learned, were not considered good patients.

He reported his observation to the nurse. She tapped his tummy with her fingers. Then she listened to it with her stethoscope.

"You need to have a bowel movement," she said.

Fusswood was quite relieved at this news. He asked her to help him to the bathroom.

"Oh, no," she replied. "Your orders say bed rest only. We don't want to put too much strain on your incision. I'll get you a bedpan."

The thought of trying to empty his bowels while lying flat

on his back made Fusswood shudder. Then he remembered.

"When Dr. Conger came in today, he told me it was time to get up. Said it was good for my lungs. I'm sure a stroll to the bathroom was just the kind of thing he had in mind. And I'll bet my incision would be much happier with me relaxing on the toilet instead of straining on the bedpan."

"Mrs. Trotter did say something in morning report about Dr. Conger suggesting that you should ambulate. But there wasn't anything written in the orders. So he must have wanted you to wait until tomorrow."

"Perhaps he forgot."

She frowned. "Dr. Conger is a very busy man, but he would never forget to write an order. Now be a good dear and use the pan."

After struggling unsuccessfully with his tormentor for half an hour, Fusswood gave up, and the nurse administered an enema. Then she brought him a small tray containing two jelly beans, a glass of chalk, and a tablespoon of sand.

"This is to help regulate your bowels," the nurse explained.

As Fusswood lay in his bed and nibbled at his intestinal hors d'oeuvres, he reflected upon the body that had served him so faithfully for the past thirty-nine years. Why had it failed him now? Was it ready for the scrap heap? Or had he been guilty of neglect? Fusswood had never paid much attention to his internal workings. He wondered if now might be time to reevaluate his laissez-faire philosophy.

Fusswood had many more opportunities for such reflections before going home. His hospitalization was a prolonged one, complicated by pneumonia, a toxic reaction to antibiotics, and a stress ulcer. By the time Fusswood was ready for discharge, he was a changed man. He pounded his still painful scar with a touch of pride, thanked me profusely for my efforts, and gave the nurses a large box of chocolates.

When Fusswood came into the office for his follow-up visit, I got a urine sample. It showed a trace of blood.

"Better check it out, Doc," he said without hesitation. "Never can tell what it might be."

9

Hiram is the last of the Stedrocks, the sole surviving representative of the descendants of Ephrain Stedrock, who in 1755 cleared two hundred acres of reluctant farmland along the brook that was to bear his name, built a house from the stones that were his first harvest, and then planted his seed. His wife, Mary, was equally hardy. She tilled the land Ephrain had cleared, kept the house he built, and tended the seed he had sown — five sons and a daughter — until the last, a sixth son, died during childbirth and became one of the two original settlers of the Stedsville Cemetery on Goreham Hill, the other being Mary. They took the place of honor at the head of a long row of Stedrocks, he identified by a small flat stone, which read:

Unnamed Infant Son of Ephrain Stedrock
b. July 17, 1764
d. July 17, 1764

and she with an upright slate, upon which was inscribed:

Mary Stedrock
1729–1764
Relic of Ephrain Stedrock
She Served the Lord, and Now She Rests

Mary Stedrock had given the clan a reproductive momentum that ought to have kept the name alive forever, but an unfortunate succession of daughters and bachelor sons depleted the Stedrock capital until only Hiram was left.

Strictly speaking, there are two other Stedrocks: Hiram and Rachel's twin boys. However, nobody counts them. When the time had come for them to make their grand entrance onto life's stage, there were some technical difficulties. It was ten o'clock at night, and Rachel, having gotten up at dawn to milk the cows and helped with haying most of the day — her only break being to make dinner for the men — was dead tired. She didn't have any energy left for one more chore. Consequently, she was not of much use when the boys needed assistance. And neither was Jenny Webster, the midwife, who couldn't do much more than shine a flashlight at them to point the way while they fought to see who would get out first. This meant that the whole business took a lot longer than it should have, and when the twins grew up to the stage where you could tell if everything was entirely there, it was apparent that a substantial amount had been left behind.

After he got the farm going, Ephrain Stedrock made a sawmill. Powered by the energy of Sted Brook, the mill had both a saw and a grinding stone, enabling Ephrain to provide the surrounding farmers with lumber, flour, and cider. The community that sprang up around Ephrain's mill was called Stedsville. The boundaries of Stedsville were defined not by geography, but by its sphere of influence, so that the farmer who went to Ephrain for cutting his lumber or milling his grain, instead of to George Barclay's mill ten miles west, was considered a Stedsvillian rather than a Barclay's Miller.

The mill attracted other settlers into the area. In the early 1800s, Stedsville was a thriving community of about a thousand souls. But by the end of the century, the Stedrock Mill,

like most of Vermont's small industries, gave way to larger
and more efficient operations in the cities. The people followed suit, and eventually the mantle as Stedsville's domi-
nant institution passed from Ephrain's Mill to the place on
Goreham Hill.

Stedsville is about five miles from Dumster. It is connected to the town by a dirt road that runs from the end of
Hill Street to a place called Center of Town. In Ephrain's
day Center of Town contained the mill, a dozen or so
homes, a church, a one-room schoolhouse, and a milk shed.
Today, only the cemetery and the Stedrock House remain.
From Center of Town, four winding roads disperse, like
frayed ends of a rope, into the surrounding hills. Actually,
the relationship between the roads and Center of Town is
just the opposite, since Center of Town is the destination,
not the origin, of these byways, which follow, both in direction and in style, the headwaters of Sted Brook. They start
as scattered ruts, abandoned logging trails, and tendencies
toward clearings, and they flow more or less downhill until
they meet near some structure that might be visited by a
vehicle, like a sugaring house or a hunting camp. Then,
having formed actual roads, they gradually coalesce until
they all merge at Center of Town. At this point, the now
unified road accompanies Sted Brook to the outskirts of
Dumster, where it crosses the brook on a bridge, which the
brook — just to show who is in charge — washes out every
few years.

Dumster suffers from a chronic sense of inferiority. It is
not big enough to be a true metropolis, and not sufficiently
quaint to be the kind of town that Flatlanders would visit,
where they could stay at the Dumster Inn, a lovely old
Victorian place with spacious rooms and tea at four; the
kind of town with stores to browse in, where there was nice
music playing, and the employees wore shirts with the name

of the store embroidered on them to help you if you were so distracted looking at all the wonderful things that you forgot to whom you should write the check; stores where you could find the perfect something for doing that task that you had never realized there was a something to do it with, like peeling avocados or removing splinters from firewood — a something you could hardly wait to get home and try out, but that, having used it once, you never used quite as much as you thought, because finding it and getting it set up and cleaning it afterward took more time than the task itself.

But Dumster doesn't have a Dumster Inn. It has the Dumster Motel, whose architectural style is Neoplywood, and whose featured attraction is cable TV. And it has Smith's Top-Notch Hardware. You don't browse in Smith's. When you walk in the door, the clerk asks you what you want. You tell him, often providing a sample of the thing in question, because most of the time it is a replacement kind of thing, and he goes and gets it for you — unless it is a complicated case, in which case Ben Smith, who is out back, is consulted and looks it over and tells you whether you can use something he has in stock as a substitute, or whether he will have to order it from Boston.

Once the selectmen, in an attack of progressivity, tried to entice a movie theater to locate in Dumster, offering as incentive to shovel the sidewalk for them, but the deal fell through. The best Dumster could do for excitement was a pizza parlor that changed owners every six months, and was then three months in renovation, so that a person could not even count on the availability of pizza in an emergency.

For serious shopping, Dumsterians have to drive two hours to The Mall in Manchester, New Hampshire. Although no Dumsterian would ever be so frivolous as to spend a night away from home just to go shopping, by a remarkable coincidence, many residents of Dumster have relatives in the Manchester area, and they often visit them in the spring at Easter and in the summer before school starts.

This is not to say that Dumsterians are not loyal to their town. They love Dumster dearly. But the townspeople have been around enough to know that on the train of urban travel, Dumster had purchased a seat in second class.

Except for people like Hiram Stedrock. For Hiram, Dumster is not just the Big Apple, it is the Only Apple. When Hiram Stedrock goes out to eat, it is to Nat's Lunch. And when he goes on a shopping spree, it is to Contremond's or Smith's. Everything else he orders from Sears. Hiram Stedrock would no more consider driving to Manchester than he would think about buying a Cuisinart. Although there might be a pair of pants in Manchester that would be better or cheaper than those at Contremond's, Hiram doesn't see the point in spending a whole day doing something that can be accomplished in an hour. In Hiram's eyes, time spent traveling is just plain wasted. Spinnin', he calls it. Hiram Stedrock doesn't have much use for spinnin'. Ever.

Every spring, when the snow melts and the ground thaws, the woods become a giant bowl of pudding. About a mile from Center of Town, there is a stretch where the Stedsville road passes through a low-lying marshy area. It is known as the Pit. If there has been a large runoff, the mud there often reaches two feet in depth. Whenever this happens, Hiram Stedrock drives his truck into the middle of the Pit, turns off the engine, and walks home. He knows that even if he could get through, he would have to spend so much time towing others out, and making such a mess in the process that it would take the road crew the better part of a week to repair the holes, that it isn't worth the effort to keep the road open.

Hiram doesn't get much appreciation for this community service. Some kid him about being lazy. Others complain about the truck being in the way. To the former, he doesn't say anything. And to the latter he just replies, "Keys are in the ignition."

Hiram was the last of Stedsville's farmers. He stayed when the others left, in part because he liked to farm, but mainly because staying is what he does. So Hiram Stedrock, with his two retarded sons and reclusive wife, who had not been seen outside the farmhouse in thirty years, scratched out a living with a small dairy herd, his sugar maples, and the little cash he got from fixing things, which some years was enough to get by and some wasn't. And as the years passed, and Hiram got to that stretch on the road of life where you begin to pay less attention to the scenery and more to the vehicle, people started saying that he would have to slack up, or he wouldn't be around much longer. But Hiram didn't slack up. Not because he didn't want to: because he couldn't. Every time he tested the rope that tethered him to his land, it was taut as a wire.

Until 1971. That was the year Henry Turnstill drove into his yard and asked Hiram Stedrock if he wanted to sell his farm. Hiram told Mr. Turnstill that he would never be able to make a living on it, but Henry said he didn't intend to; he just wanted to know was Hiram going to take his offer or not, because he had to get back to New York that day. It didn't take much figuring for Hiram to give his answer. Henry Turnstill gave Hiram Stedrock a check for twenty thousand dollars, and Hiram Stedrock gave Henry Turnstill title to the farmhouse, the barn, the sawmill, and two hundred acres of land, more or less, the less being one acre tucked in the back corner of the sugar-maple grove. Henry Turnstill moved into the big farmhouse by himself, while Hiram Stedrock, his family, and two cows, which he kept not so much for milk as for company, moved into a small trailer that hardly seemed big enough for one person, but that suited the four Stedrocks just fine.

Henry Turnstill came to Stedsville in a cloud of mystery. The general assumption was that he had fled New York when several of his investments, some financial, others personal, went sour. Some said he had swindled his bank of large sums of money but had escaped prosecution on a technicality. Others claimed that he was a former gangland member who had changed his name and hidden in the country to avoid assassination. Still others were sure that he was the black sheep of a wealthy New York family, who had made a hasty marriage beneath his station and left both the marriage and the station when he came to his senses. Henry Turnstill, whose only form of social contact was farm auctions, did nothing himself to dispel the cloud. It was not that he was antisocial, although he could hardly be called a social butterfly. It was just that Henry Turnstill was so obsessed with his mission that he considered any activity not contributing directly to its attainment to be an unnecessary distraction and a complete waste of time. His mission was this: to create order in an intolerably disorderly world. The place he had picked to start was one that generations of Stedrocks, in conspiracy with Nature, had thrown into such a state of disarray that even Henry at times feared he would not be able to rectify it in his lifetime.

Both Henry Turnstill and the Stedrocks were avid conservationists. However, while Henry was concerned with the preservation of things, the Stedrocks were savers of energy. If the chicken coop collapsed, it was abandoned and a new one built elsewhere. Should a tractor die in the middle of the cornfield, it was moved just far enough to keep it from being in the way. Anything that might be used someday for spare parts was saved in the spot closest to where it had last been used. The cumulative effect of this conservation policy was to produce an appearance typical of farms in Vermont. Tumbledown buildings and rusting equipment dotted the land, as if their arrangement had been determined by some Committee for the Improvement of Junkyards, which had decided that each piece should be given its own space so that its beauty and relationship to the environment could better be appreciated.

Henry Turnstill got rid of the old plows and the old tractors. He threw out the old tires. He tore down the chicken coops and the outhouses and the sheds. He gutted the farmhouse. When everything that could be was torn down, he started in on the building up. Restoration, he called it. If Hiram Stedrock had been called in as a consultant to advise Henry on what the place had looked like when his ancestors had lived there — which he never was — he might have noted that the house, when finished, with its polyurethaned floors, Williamsburg wallpaper, and Chippendale furniture, bore no discernible resemblance to the house in which he had lived for sixty-two years and his ancestors for some one hundred and fifty before that. The house, except for the addition of indoor plumbing about thirty years ago and electricity about twenty, had changed so little from its original state that it really wouldn't have needed any restoration at all in order to qualify as an historical monument — if Stedsville had a society for historical monuments.

It did. The Stedsville Historical Society, a thriving organization of twenty-five eager souls, which was founded in 1975 by Buffy Uprite and which had picked, as its first historical monument, the Stedrock farmhouse. Surprisingly, despite the importance of Stedrocks in Stedsville history, Hiram Stedrock is not a member of the Society. More surprising still, when the Society decided to have a talk on "The History of Stedsville Farms," to be followed by a tour and tea at Buffy's, it was not Hiram Stedrock they asked to speak, but a professor from Dartmouth, who came down to show slides and afterward sold autographed copies of his book, *Old Vermont Farms*. In all fairness to the Society, it would have been difficult to invite Hiram even if they had wanted to, for he didn't have any slides to show. And most of the history he could show had been restored away.

After he finished the house, Henry restored the barn. He had bought a pair of Arabian horses to add a touch of authenticity, but when he saw what they did to his polished pine flooring, he asked Hiram to keep them and recalled them only for viewing on special occasions. He even restored the old sawmill, complete with a genuine waterwheel that he got from California, and when it was installed, after Hiram Stedrock adjusted a few things that the restoration experts had overlooked, it actually worked. Because of the sawdust, Henry never used it to cut lumber, but from time to time he would open the millrun and turn on the saw just to show that he could.

Having tackled the mess made by man, Henry set to work on Nature's. He attacked the trespassing trees and, after a fierce battle, drove them back behind the stone walls, liberating the captive fields. There were heavy casualties on both sides, including Henry Turnstill himself, who almost cut off his foot with an axe the only time he actually tried to take up arms against his foe himself. He went after the hemlock stand with a vengeance, hacking away at the unruly trees until he had created row upon row of well-groomed, orderly, identical conifers, standing, like soldiers waiting for inspection, in long, straight lines, with not a single bramble to mar the needle-covered parade ground on which they stood.

The maples were next to succumb to the Turnstill juggernaut. He weeded out the old, the infirm, and the physically defective. Then he trimmed those that remained just enough for the sun to cast a little spot of light on the ground between each tree.

He saved the birches for last. Although Nature gave the birch great beauty, she did not endow it with strong ethnic roots, so that it is scattered in the forest, alone, in pairs, or occasionally in small clumps, but never in its own grove. Henry Turnstill was singularly displeased with such shabby treatment of this purest of trees, and he set about to right the wrong. At the back of the farm, the land sloped upward until it met the ridge leading to Goreham Hill. Henry began by systematically eliminating from the slope every single tree of non-Birchyan origin. Next he deported all but those members of the species that had the whitest bark and the straightest trunks, a task that required the sacrifice of a large number of otherwise healthy trees, since the birches of Stedsville had not been very well trained in either posture or grooming. Around the privileged few that were allowed to stay, every stump was uprooted, every stone removed, and every unsightly hillock leveled. Finally, adding insult to his injured enemy, he planted Kentucky bluegrass as ground cover. The result was spectacular. Each individual birch stood in splendid isolation from the others, its beauty framed magnificently by the carpet of blue-green grass lying at its feet.

People came from everywhere to admire Henry's work. Those who had money bought a piece of Stedsville so they could create their own imitation of the Turnstill masterpiece. Fields returned to the hillsides. Ponds sprang up at every spring. Manicured forests multiplied. Even a polo field appeared. Pretty soon all of Stedsville looked like Henry Turnstill's place.

I fell in love with Stedsville the first time I saw it. It was the place I skied in winter and ran in summer. It was the place I took my Flatland friends when I wanted them to see the beauty of Vermont. Unspoiled by the need to be useful, it was the kind of place that made you feel good about the

world; the kind of place that made you believe in the value
of the upper class.

Henry Turnstill was a pioneer, the first of many who
would reclaim the territory the farmers had abandoned,
allowing the forests to sneak back over the stone walls and
gobble up their fields, and the brambles to squat on every
inch of bare land that the forests left alone. They would
make a new life, not just for Stedsville, but for Hiram Stedrock, because the pioneers, although they were determined
and full of spirit, were a little lacking in experience when it
came to actual pioneering. They would need Hiram
Stedrock to show them where to dig the ponds for their
ducks. And they would need Hiram Stedrock to fix the
chimneys that were letting the winds in instead of the smoke
out. And they would need Hiram Stedrock to install all
those things that pioneers use to conquer the wilderness,
like woodstoves and hot tubs and electric fences. Hiram
Stedrock did. And did, to his amazement, for more money
than he ever thought it possible to make.

The pioneers loved Hiram Stedrock. He became a Doc
Franklin of the mechanical arts: a man who, like his medical
counterpart, was revered more for what people thought he
ought to be than for what he actually was. Hiram Stedrock
could see this quite clearly and thought it rather amusing.
But Doc Franklin, having taken himself quite seriously,
never saw it at all.

≥ *10* ⩊

*I*t *was late October.* Houses broke out in storm windows. Rototillers roamed the gardens. Woodpiles were ripening. And Hiram Stedrock put on his winter outfit. It was a red-and-black-checked wool jacket, with a cap that would have matched except that the red checks were green. It was the only hint of frivolity in his otherwise very practical life.

It was not hard to tell when Hiram Stedrock was nearby. His presence was announced by a very distinct fragrance — a blend of fresh milk, stale straw, and cow dung — which, despite its composition, was not at all unpleasant. The fragrance did not result from parsimony in Hiram Stedrock's use of the bath, for both he and his animals were quite clean, but from years of cohabitation with his herd of Guernseys, which had created a kind of olfactory homeostasis, so that he smelled slightly like a cow, and the cows wore a subtle but definite Odeur de Hiram.

Hiram Stedrock did not have much of a medical record. When something went wrong with his body he usually fixed it himself. I read the last entry. It was dated August 25, 1974. Hiram Stedrock had cut his leg with a chain saw. He had tried unsuccessfully to treat it with Bag Balm and duct tape, the former being his standard remedy for any defect in the integument, and the latter his favorite material for patching a leak. Doc Franklin's note was typically succinct:

> Tried to make his leg into kindling.
> Damn near did.
> Forty-two stitches.

When I entered the room, Hiram acknowledged my presence with a short but courteous nod.

"Good morning, Mr. Stedrock," I said. "Some weather we're having." This was my favorite icebreaker. Vermonters enjoy talking about weather. It's easy. On a good day, you could make an observation about the weather every hour without fear of repeating yourself.

Hiram Stedrock nodded but said nothing. Meteorology was apparently not one of his hobbies. I tried again.

"Roads looked pretty good today." Although this is usually a winter topic, often used as a follow-up to weather, I figured with winter so close at hand it was acceptable.

Hiram shrugged. His face took on a slightly pained expression.

"How's your wood?"

Vermont men are a very religious lot. Pantheists, mostly. Every summer they build a giant altar to their god. It is constructed entirely of small pieces of wood. In winter they burn the altar. The preparation of their altar is a ritual of sacrifice, the burning an act of redemption. No Vermonter can resist an offer to expound upon his woodpile.

Hiram's mouth quivered slightly as if it were about to open, but no words came out. He squirmed restlessly in his seat. Hiram Stedrock did not like questions, especially ones that could not be answered without a simple nod or a grunt. Like all Stedrocks, Hiram believed that his brain had been stocked in utero with a finite supply of words, and that he was expected to ration this stockpile to meet his lifetime communication needs. Hiram Stedrock lived in constant dread that someday he might get into a desperate situation, only to find out in midsentence that he had squandered his allotment with too many passings of the time of day.

Rebuffed in my attempts at casual conversation, I decided to get down to business.

"Well, Mr. Stedrock, what seems to be the problem today?"

"Don't know."

I was pretty fluent by now in the native tongue, but occasionally I slipped up. Vermont is a literal language. By asking Hiram Stedrock what his problem was, I had asked him to render a diagnosis. That was my job. I corrected my error.

"Something must be bothering you a great deal for you to come to the doctor. If you tell me what it is, I might be able to help you."

"It's private."

"I'm afraid that doesn't help me much."

"It's *real* private!" he said, wincing as he added *real.* The wasted word hurt.

"I see," I replied.

I didn't see at all, but since Hiram appeared reluctant to amplify upon this statement, I would have to try another approach.

"I'm afraid that's not quite enough information for me to make a diagnosis, Mr. Stedrock. This is what I suggest we do. I will leave the room. You will turn your chair around and discuss your problem with the wall until you feel comfortable talking about it. When you're ready, knock on the door, and I'll come back."

Beads of sweat broke out on Hiram's forehead. The prospect of spending a substantial share of his vocabular reserves on a wall terrified him. There was no choice but to fess up.

"It don't work."

"What don't work?"

"It!"

Under conventional rules of English grammar, *it* is classified as an indefinite pronoun. However, when used by a male patient talking to his doctor, the meaning is quite definite indeed.

Hiram was suffering from Male Troubles.

SERIOUS READER NOTE: Troubles of the female have had a long and illustrious career in the annals of medical symptomatology. Countless volumes have been written on the subject, and the number of nostrums designed for their cure is legion. Female Troubles is a distinguished affliction. It is suitable for discussion at even the most proper of public gatherings.

Not so Male Troubles. Long has it wallowed in the backwaters of unwanted diseases. Should a man try to talk about his Troubles in public, he will soon find himself, like Hiram almost did, talking to the wall.

Inability to be open about their Troubles has had dire consequences for men. Forced to suppress the need to share their feelings about their sexuality, they have pretended to be insensitive and unfeeling. Unable to learn from their peers, they have been condemned to ignorance about their most intimate body parts. For example, it is a commonly held belief among men that the penis, although connected to the body by the normal complement of nerves, blood vessels, and the like, is a completely independent organism equipped with its own power supply and capable of being activated on command by the simple flick of a switch.

Nothing, of course, could be further from the truth. The penis is very much a mainstream organ — so much so, that if any one of the others should suffer the slightest malaise, it will become paralyzed with concern and be unable to carry out its assigned duties.

The penis is a sensitive organ. It is, therefore, very vulnerable to criticism. If a man says anything derogatory about his penis, or if he even thinks about it in critical terms, it will curl up and sulk.

The penis is also extremely shy. It does not like attention. A watched penis never rises.

Usually men do not learn these truths until late in life. When they do, they think something is wrong. This invariably brings them scurrying to the doctor.

My job in such a case is to explain to the patient that if he devotes less attention to the state of It, and more to the state of himself, It will usually take care of Itself.

"Do not be alarmed, Hiram. What you have noticed is a completely normal phenomenon: a temporary malfunction caused by some minor upset in your life, like a sick cow, or a spat with your wife, or perhaps a touch of the flu."

Hiram was puzzled. In his view of life, there were only two states: fixed and broke. The fixed things needed only a little maintenance to keep going, while the broke ones either had to be fixed or discarded.

Teaching Hiram Stedrock to listen to his body could be difficult. Nonetheless, I had to try.

"Think of your penis as a weathervane," I said. "It tells you which way the winds of your body are blowing. When you are up, so is it, and when you're down, well . . ." I stopped here, wondering how much more explicit I should be.

Hiram shook his head. "Ain't."

I tried again.

"I know this is hard to believe, but the fact is that your ability to have an erection can be affected by the slightest thing. The penis is a very delicate organ."

"Ain't it," he repeated.

"Pardon?" Now it was my turn to be confused.

"When you piss, and you shake It to stop the drip, so you can put It away . . ." Hiram stopped and looked at me expectantly, hoping that he had provided sufficient data for me to fix It without further discussion. He hadn't.

"Yes?"

"No."

"No?"

"It don't."

"It don't what?"

"It don't stop."

Finally I understood. The problem was not his penis. It was his prostate. The prostate is a small gland that sits right where the bladder empties into the penis. Its job is to produce the milky fluid that renders more hospitable to sperm the stream in which they travel as they make their way from testis to outside world. For no apparent reason, the gland gets bigger with age. Because of its location, an enlarged prostate can effectively gum up the waterworks, making it hard for a man to pee when he so desires and hard to stop when he is done.

I explained all this to Hiram as succinctly as possible.

"Can you fix it?" he asked.

"I can't, but Dr. Flushing can. She's our urologist, a medical plumber. She takes a small scraper, inserts it through your penis up to the prostate, and then trims off the excess tissue."

"Like a Roto-Rooter."

"Exactly. It's a simple operation. Hardly any risk. Sometimes, however, you do lose control of urination altogether."

"Have to?"

SERIOUS READER NOTE: It was reasonable that Hiram, who was not particularly enthusiastic about having his plumbing revised, would want to know if the proposed surgery was really necessary. He had no way of knowing that this is just the kind of question that people who like to harass doctors love to ask — like people who work for the government and have nothing better to do than to complain that we perform unnecessary operations, order unnecessary tests, and prescribe unnecessary treatments; people who, when it comes to unnecessariness, are definitely in glass houses.

The answer to his question is no. He could let his prostate grow without any dire consequences. There is considerable discretion as to when to trim a prostate. When Dr. Flushing first arrived at Emmeline Talbot Memorial Hospital, she could hardly find a prostate that didn't need to be shorter on the sides or have a little taken off the top. But now that her practice is more established, and she is kept pretty busy covering four different hospitals, she prefers to let them grow a bit longer before cutting.

Whether the operation is necessary is not the point. A house with no furniture serves perfectly well as shelter. A person could survive on soybeans and brewer's yeast alone. And you can get perfectly clean without a hot tub. You could probably even do pretty well without a doctor. So what? If life were to be rid of all its superfluities, we could probably be done with it in about fifteen years. And nobody would complain when it was over.

"Deciding when to have your prostate surgery is like deciding when to paint your house," I explained. "You can do

III

it when the first sign of flaking appears, or you can wait until the wood is bare and the boards are beginning to warp. It's up to you."

"Guess I'll wait," said Hiram. "Never was much for paintin'."

11

I said in the introduction that I was writing this diary because my mother asked me to. It is true that my mother was the person who specifically mentioned the project. She also gave me many useful suggestions, like what topics I should cover, and what I should wear for my picture on the back cover. She even gave me several books by James Herriot, an English veterinarian who wrote about his practice in the hills of Yorkshire. She thought he would be a good role model, animals being a lot like people, and hills being hills, whether they are in Vermont or Yorkshire.

But the actual inspiration, which I would have mentioned in the dedication but didn't because I was afraid it might cause some family friction, came from my mother's sister, Aunt Helen.

My mother and Aunt Helen were raised in Kokomo, Indiana. Their father, George Canfield, owned a factory in Kokomo that made toilet seats: Canfield Seat Company. Although it was a small company, Canfield toilet seats were highly regarded. The company specialized in personalized toilet seats, and its top-of-the-line model, the Custom Fit, was world famous. Each Custom Fit seat was individually cast from a mold so as to conform precisely to the anatomy of the customer, and the lids were hand-decorated by artists under exclusive contract to Canfield Seat Company. A Custom Fit was not just a toilet seat. It was a work of art. The most famous Canfield Custom Fit was the one Grandpa Canfield made for Greta Garbo. It was electrically heated — the first of its kind — and on the lid was a picture of Greta that was studded with one hundred and twenty diamonds. Grandpa Canfield was very proud of this seat. On the mantelpiece in Grandma and Grandpa Canfield's home was a picture of Grandpa holding the toilet seat in one hand and a picture of Greta in the other.

The Canfield Seat Company was one of Kokomo's distinguished institutions. My Aunt Helen, however, never fully appreciated the family business. Whenever someone asked what her father did, she replied, "He's in manufacturing," and quickly changed the subject.

The reason Aunt Helen was unable to give much respect or admiration to her father's business was that she had already spent it all on her Uncle Ned. Uncle Ned was a doctor. He also lived in Kokomo and had two boys who were about the same age as my mother and Helen. The four were good friends and often traveled around town together. Wherever they went, people would stop them and say to the boys, "Aren't you Dr. Canfield's boys? You're so lucky to have him for a father. He's a wonderful man, you know."

The boys didn't know this at all: they hardly ever saw their father. He was usually off saving lives or being admired for what a wonderful person he was. But they didn't particularly mind his absence from the family nest, because when he did come home, he spent most of his time in his favorite chair, puffing on his pipe, reading his medical journals, and complaining about how tired he was. His only interaction with the family occurred when he interrupted these pursuits to give orders to his wife for correction of the bad habits his children had developed under her negligent supervision. He treated her just like one of the nurses at the hospital, and she never told him what she thought of his behavior, which was that they were supposed to be partners in this business of having a family, and that if he didn't have anything useful to contribute, at least he could keep his mouth shut.

Uncle Ned's greatest paternal fear was that his children would grow up to be wimps. He was constantly on the alert for any signs that his children were developing tendencies in this direction, especially when it came to being sick.

In a normal family, the balance of power is heavily tipped in favor of parents. Children have little with which to defend themselves from the barrage of parental artillery, but there is one weapon that is particularly effective, and kids rely upon it frequently when the shelling gets especially heavy: the stomach ache.

A child who complains of a stomach ache can ordinarily expect a temporary reprieve from any impending punishment and a modicum of parental sympathy. If he is lucky, he might even get a little spoiling thrown in. In Uncle Ned's house, what a child got was the Inquisition.

First came the Interrogation. "Where is the pain? When did it start? Is it sharp or is it dull?" These are questions no kid has the slightest idea how to answer, since to the kid, a stomach ache is not a particular pain existing at an actual point in time and space, but a metaphysical concept, a statement of how he feels about the world.

Next was the Examination. Uncle Ned would poke and prod and pound the little tummy until he was satisfied that he had beaten the imposter into submission. And should any doubts still remain as to what was going on, the coup de grace was delivered by his favorite instrument of diagnostic torture: the rectal thermometer. He obtained therefrom proof beyond any shadow of a reasonable doubt that the child in question was guilty as charged of impersonating an illness.

Finally, the Sentence. Delivering ominous threats about what happened to people who went to the doctor when there was nothing wrong with them, Uncle Ned dispatched the now subjugated child to a term of hard labor at whichever of his particular chores was the most despised. Uncle Ned never explained exactly what became of such malingerers. This may have been out of deference to those of his patients who also fell into this category, the ones who were largely responsible for the success of his practice. But his tone implied that it was pretty awful.

It was quite a performance to behold, a grown man marshaling all his powers of intimidation on an unhappy child. And very effective.

It was so effective that when Billy, the older of his two boys, got a stomach ache, no one knew about it until his mother found him hiding in the closet with a temperature of one hundred and four, mumbling deliriously, "Tummy OK! Tummy OK!" Fortunately his father was not home at the time. The surgeon said it was the worst case of appendicitis he had ever seen. That made Uncle Ned very proud. When asked how it was that a doctor's kid had almost died from appendicitis, he replied, "Tough little kid, that Billy. Never complains."

None of this mattered to Helen. She worshipped her uncle, and he, in turn, gave her the love that by birthright belonged to his own children. When Uncle Ned died, he left Helen his medical books and said in his will that he hoped someday she would be able to give them to children of her own.

Helen was determined that her son would grow up to be a doctor. When her only child turned out to be a daughter, she was heartbroken. When this daughter graduated summa cum laude from Indiana University, went on to be first in her class at Stanford Business School, and later founded a very successful company that designed irrigation systems for Third World countries, she was unmoved. Only after a story appeared about her in *Time,* and all the neighbors congratulated her, did she allow herself to be slightly consoled.

Just as Uncle Ned had crossed family lines to bestow his parental affection, so did Aunt Helen give to me the attention that should have been reserved for her daughter. On my fifth birthday she gave me a toy doctor's kit. In college she sent me a box of homemade chocolate chip cookies every week for four years. And for my college graduation, she passed on to me the treasured copy of *Gray's Anatomy* that she had received from Uncle Ned.

I liked Aunt Helen. I could confide in her without fear of being criticized. And she was always full of praise for even the slightest of my accomplishments. When I went home for holidays, I always paid her a visit.

On such occasions, there was one question she always asked me. As many times as she had asked it before, she never seemed to tire of hearing the answer. And I never tired of giving it.

"What does it take to be a doctor?"

"That's a hard question to answer," I would always start. "The years of training and long work hours require tremendous dedication. In order to understand the complexities of medical science, a person must have a keen intellect. Then there is the responsibility of holding a human life in your hands and knowing that the slightest misstep or hesitation can spell the difference between life and death. For that, a doctor needs to be bold and decisive, while at the same time remaining calm and collected. But" — at this point I would pause briefly to indicate the importance of what I was about to say — "even if someone has all of these abilities, they will be of no use to him unless he also is driven by a burning desire to achieve the impossible."

It was a moving speech for both of us. A dreamy look would come over Aunt Helen's face as she contemplated what might have been had her sister died unexpectedly and left a little nephew for her to raise. And I would feel uplifted, transported by an awareness of how wonderful it was to be a doctor. It was a remarkable feeling, much like that a preacher must get when, in the midst of a particularly inspiring sermon, he gazes out over his congregation and, seeing the reverent looks on their faces, realizes that he truly is a Messenger of God.

The speech had only one shortcoming. It was not entirely accurate. It did not mention the one virtue so crucial to being a doctor that without it none of us could ever perform our routine miracles.

Arrogance.

———————————◄►►———————————

SERIOUS READER NOTE: Arrogance is the sine qua non, the ne plus ultra, the there-but-for-the-grace-of-God-go-I, of doctoring. For reasons I have never understood, arrogance is not one of the more popular virtues. More than any of the other qualities that distinguish men from animals, it is arrogance that has been responsible for the advancement of the human race. Why else would it be found in greatest abundance among those who have the most important positions in society?

Medical educators have long recognized the importance of arrogance in the practice of medicine. They take great pains to ensure that those who are admitted to medical school are well endowed with an ample supply. This they accomplish by the simple expedient of making medical school as expensive as possible, thereby ensuring that students come from the wealthy, where arrogance is a birth-right, or are those of the lower classes who have acquired sufficient arrogance to muscle in on credit.

Native arrogance, however, must be multiplied many times over before it is adequate to serve a doctor's needs. Even then it is not ready. Like any source of power, arrogance is useless unless it can be harnessed. This is the purpose of medical school. Think of the physician as a mighty eagle. The medical student is a baby eaglet. And medical school is the nest in which the eaglet will be nurtured until it is ready to go out on its own.

Like all newborns, the students are hungry when first they arrive at school, but their delicate little tummies are not yet ready for the rich diet that will be used to promote their growth. Patiently the professors whisper to them in a magical new tongue. Eagerly the students mimic it, and the soothing words still their cries of hunger. But words alone give little sustenance. Accordingly, during their first year, students are gradually introduced to the food of knowledge. Generous help-ings of pharmacology and physiology, small portions of physical diagnosis, and an occasional morsel of surgery are administered under the watchful eyes of their professors, who are constantly alert for any signs of malnutrition or overfeeding.

By the end of their second year, they are ready to try their first excursion from the nest. Dressed in white coats and carrying little black bags, the fledglings are quite cute as they waddle around the hospital behind their professors, jabbering excitedly and stopping from time to time at a bedside to try out their new toys. They look so much like real doctors that a casual observer might be deceived. But they are not. Deep down inside, their souls still harbor the doubts and fears of ordinary mortals.

At four years of age, they are ready to leave the nest for good. In the year that follows — the internship — the budding young healers finish their upbringing under the tutelage of teachers who have been specially trained to help them through the final phases of their education. These teachers inspire them to greater heights, first by instructing them, then by agreeing with them, and at last by sub-

mitting to them. They carefully mark the progress of their charges by the interns' transition from at first asking, then to discussing, and finally to ordering.

But more important than the instruction interns receive from their nurses is the attention they are given. Interns get precious little of this vital substance during this stage of their training. Especially from patients. When a patient leaves the hospital, it is not the intern he remembers and wants to thank for saving his life. It is his "real" doctor. She is the one whose name is engraved on his little plastic wristband. She is also the one whose name is on the piece of paper the patient gets that tells him how much it cost to have his life saved. Souvenirs like this help a patient remember who his real doctor is, even if she didn't have much to do with saving the patient's actual life, being, as real doctors often are, so busy saving lives in general that they don't have time to save any one particular life.

Were it not for the nurses' constant reminders of how wonderful he is, treatment like this could render an intern susceptible to an attack of humility. Even the mildest case of this dread affliction would almost certainly prevent him from reaching the pinnacle of his education: residency.

Among the residents, one stands out above all the others: the surgical chief resident. For sheer magnificence, he is truly without equal. Watch him as he swoops down to the bedside of some poor Life whose failing heart has just given its last beat. Extending his hand palm upward to the assembled flock, he accepts the proffered blade. Without hesitation, he plunges the knife deep into the chest and, in one mighty slash, lays it open, exposing the defective organ. With his bare hands he grasps the inert heart and begins to squeeze. Energized by the power in his hands, the stagnant blood begins to flow, and the Life, which had been given up for dead, is miraculously restored. No less majestic is he when some minutes later the Life, having had the opportunity to show its appreciation for reprieve, humbly requests permission to retire from the scene. Nodding once to indicate that the request has been granted, the chief withdraws his hand and flies off in search of another Life to save.

The chief resident demands respect, but he does not inspire adulation. That is a privilege reserved for the premier of the species, the mature adult male. Easily identified by the telltale shock of white hair, he is a truly elegant bird. His feathers have been smoothed by the winds of time, and his talons, blunted from years of grabbing death's stony ground, are no longer dangerous. He looks more the protector than the predator; a source of comfort, not a cause for fear. When perched he appears almost tame.

───────── ◄•► ─────────

Doc Franklin was a good example. Though I knew him only briefly, I think about him often. I wonder if my patients will worship me the way they do him. Not for a long time, I suspect. But I know my time will come. I just hope it will be in my own lifetime.

12

Maple Street comes to a dead end at the back of the Old North Church cemetery. The last house on the right is a Queen Anne Victorian with a turret on top and a large balcony overlooking the cemetery. A flower-bordered cobblestone path leads from the wrought-iron gate through a perfectly groomed lawn up to the porch. On the porch is one of those old-fashioned swing sofas, the kind that is just right for watching the performance of a warm summer evening. The front door is solid oak. On it is a brass knocker in the shape of a lion's head and a placard that reads 1811, the year in which the house was built. The door announces to all that, should they chance to step through its portals, they would find within a world of elegance. And so they should: spacious rooms with tall ceilings and long, thin windows; an open, winding staircase to the second floor; polished hardwood floors; in the living room, a large marble fireplace; and in the kitchen, a brick hearth.

"The perfect home for a doctor," said the realtor. I fell in love with it the first time I saw it. I could hardly wait until Trine came out and I could show it to her. I had no doubt she would be impressed with my selection for the family home. I was right. One look was all it took.

"You want it," she said, "you clean it!"

We bought the house across the street. It is an ordinary Cape with a nice yard, which, as Trine reminds me once a week, would hold a swimming pool very nicely, and it is very comfortable. It is also easy to clean. It's the perfect house for us. Of course, it's not actually ours. Not yet, anyway. It belongs to Dorothy Partridge. It became Mrs. Partridge's house when she sold it to us, at which time she acquired title to what had formerly been the Bugbee place. When Walter Bugbee, who had built the house, lived there, it was known as the house on the Talbot property, having been part of the Talbot estate until Bugbee bought the half-acre from John Wilbur Talbot in 1953. This is not unusual. Nobody in Vermont lives in his own house. Until he leaves it.

The walk from Mrs. Partridge's house to the hospital is quite nice: down Maple Street to Hill and then up Hill to the turnoff for Bill Easton's farm. But there is a much better route to take if weather permits. Across from the hospital are woods that extend all the way down to the cemetery. Constructed by the kids of Dumster as a shortcut to the Sted Brook swimming hole, a footpath traverses these woods. About halfway to the cemetery, the path crosses the top of a small knoll from which there is a spectacular view of Dumster, the Connecticut River, and the New Hampshire hills beyond.

It was six o'clock in the evening and the sun had retired for the night, but a full moon and yesterday's snowfall provided more than ample illumination as I headed home. December twentieth — six months to the day since my arrival in Dumster. I stopped at the knoll. The moon, perfectly framed between the snow-laden trees, hung suspended over the distant hills and cast eerie reflections on the ground in front of me. The time and the place were quite conducive to philosophical observations about my new life. But I had forgotten my jacket, so I put my contemplations on hold and hurried on home.

Being Thursday, it was Trine's turn to cook. Warm, suppery smells greeted me as I opened the door. There was a flurry of activity in the kitchen. Everyone was just getting ready to sit down at the table. Suppertime was my favorite part of the day. Not because of the food. Because of Family Report. For Family Report, each member selected the one event from the day that he or she considered to be of greatest general interest and presented it to the rest of the family for their edification and amusement. Report proceeded in chronological order. Nadya was first. She described in great detail the snowman she had made with her friends. It was her first. I complimented her on her achievement.

Dylan was next. "You'll never believe what happened today, Daddy," she began. "I was walking home after school, and Robert Redford drove up in a silver Mercedes convertible with red velvet seats. He asked me if I wanted a ride. OK, I know what you and Mommy said about not taking rides from strangers. But Robert Redford? I mean, what would you do? So I got in. Well, you wouldn't believe this car. It was, like, so utterly awesome, it was . . . moldation! There was a TV on the dashboard, and a place to hold drinks, and the seat was heated. (I thought I had peed in my pants — I was *soooo* embarrassed.) So Robert Redford turns to me and he goes, 'How would you like to be in the movies?' And then he drove along, and you know what happened? We were in Hollywood. And Robert goes, 'Well, I gotta go now, but I'll see you when we start shooting. Oh, by the way, you can keep the car.' Then he kissed me on the cheek and left."

"Thank you, Dilly," said Trine. "That was a very interesting report."

"You're welcome, Mommy," said Nadya. At the time of

our exodus from California, Julie, Trine, and I had to figure out what to do with Matthew and Dylan. We let them decide for themselves. Matthew opted for a new life in the country, but Dylan preferred to stay with her mother. Nadya, who maintains telepathic communication with her half sister, gives Dylan's report each night.

"Hot lunch was pizza," said Matt.

Trine told us that her estate tax examination was absolutely impossible. She was sure she had failed it miserably. Nobody was surprised. Trine, by her own account, had failed almost half her courses in law school. Despite this abysmal performance, she had somehow managed to make the top 10 percent of her class. Trine never explained this discrepancy to me. I figured it had something to do with being a foreigner.

Finally it was my turn. My usual source of information for Report was Maggie, who was a gold mine of hospital gossip. Today she had given me the news that Carl Cutterup had a new girlfriend. Since this was the third such report on Dr. Cutterup in the last four weeks, I elected to discuss instead a patient who, I was pretty sure, would be of interest to the family.

"I saw Eleanor Contremond today." Nadya's ears perked up at the mention of this name. Eleanor Contremond was the mother of Darlene Contremond, her best friend.

"How come?" asked Trine.

"She's been feeling run-down lately. I think it's probably —"

"Her husband," interjected Trine. "That's what it is. It was bound to happen." When in doubt, which was rarely, Trine always blamed a wife's problems on having a husband for a spouse.

"I don't think that's what it is," I protested. "After all, every marriage has a husband. Even ours."

"I know."

"I suspect there's something else going on. She looks a wreck — feels it too. Can't sleep. Can't do her work. And always snapping at her kids. I think she might have an underactive thyroid. I ordered some tests. They should come back by Monday. Then we'll see."

"Hmpf," she snorted. "That's a waste of time."

"I wouldn't say that."

"You already did. You told me yourself that never has one symptom cost so much to so little end as a case of the blahs."

SERIOUS READER NOTE: Trine was right. Being tired is rarely a sign of disease. I don't know how many times I have told this to some patient who is convinced that he is hopelessly afflicted with some terrible disease just because he can't seem to get up in the morning like he used to, and who, when I have finished my pitch, responds with something like, "Well, that's easy for you to say, but my cousin was feeling just the way I do, and he went to his doctor, and the doctor did some tests and found out that he had what would have been a very serious case of something-or-otheritis, if the doctor hadn't discovered it just in the nick of time."

Quite possibly the patient is correct. A tired person could certainly be sick. But if there is a disease lurking in the background, something else will be wrong: loss of weight, fever, persistent cough, or nagging pain. Without any such symptoms, the chances that even the nosiest of doctors will ferret out an internal malfunction are pretty slim.

Not that we shouldn't try. After all, nothing ventured, nothing gained. You never can tell what might pop up when you cast your diagnostic net into the sea. But in the case of fatigue, the catch is invariably the inedible red herring.

Being tired is a warning light on the dashboard of life. It's an indication that the time has come for a change, any change: a new breakfast cereal, a new hobby, a new book, a new spouse — anything except a new pill.

This is not to say someone who has lost his get-up-and-go shouldn't make one last effort to get up and go to see his doctor. We can be helpful in selecting the life-style modification best suited to a person's taste and pocketbook or in resolving intrafamilial disputes over how much sympathy the tired one is entitled to receive. Besides, whenever a question begins "Should I go to the doctor if . . . ?," the answer is always yes.

"I'm just making sure," I rebutted lamely. "Besides, what would she think if I didn't order any tests?"

"She'd think you were being honest," retorted Trine. "I suppose you also suggested a heavy dose of your standard remedy when you can't find anything wrong? To turn off her warning light on the dashboard of life?"

"Of course not," I lied. "Eleanor's not the jogging type. What I told her was that if her tests came out OK, it might be a good idea for her to take up a hobby."

"Golf, perhaps? Or maybe hunting?"

"I didn't mention those particular activities, but if one of them appealed to her, I would certainly encourage her to pursue it."

"Brilliant doctor strikes again! Just what she needs. Another have-to. As if being married to a husband wasn't enough."

"Jim isn't a bad husband," I replied, making one last effort to stem the tide of her argument, although I feared it had already acquired sufficient momentum to carry it to conclusion without any further assistance on my part. "You said so yourself."

"No, he's not a bad husband. Ted Kennedy isn't a bad politician. Frank Sinatra isn't a bad singer. And Al Capone wasn't a bad gangster. But what kind of wives would they make? Can you imagine Jim Contremond ironing his own shirts? Hah!"

This last question, appearing to be of a rhetorical nature, gave me a much-needed opportunity to change the subject, which I did. But I resolved to take a different approach next time I saw Eleanor.

When she came back for her follow-up appointment, Eleanor looked even worse. Tincture of time had not helped.

"Tell me what your typical day is like," I asked her after we had gone over her laboratory tests, which, as Trine had predicted, were normal.

"I get up at five to fix breakfast for Jim and make his lunch. Then I get the kids up and feed them. After Darlene gets the bus, I take Billy to the baby-sitter and go to work. I get out of work at four-thirty, pick up Billy, and, unless I have shopping to do, come home to start dinner. After the kids are in bed, I try to do something relaxing, like ironing or sewing. I like to get to bed before eleven, so that Jim and I can talk a little. But usually he's tired, and he falls asleep as soon as he hits the pillow, or right after he finishes . . ." She hesitated awkwardly. I think she was about to say "with me" but changed to "making love."

"What about weekends?"

"I clean the house on Saturday. Sunday morning we go to church, and after that I fix Sunday dinner, if it's my turn."

"You and Jim share cooking responsibilities?" I was amazed. Jim Contremond came from a long line of Vermont males who consider cooking to be some kind of sex-linked disease. Even this modest sign of male liberation was pleasantly surprising. Perhaps times really were changing.

"Not exactly." Eleanor smiled at what she thought was intended as a humorous remark. "Madeline and I alternate. One week she and Dan come over to our place, and the next we go over there. That gives us each a break."

"Good idea. That gives you every other Sunday afternoon completely free. What do you usually do?"

She shrugged. "Nothing much."

"Well, then, why don't you ask Jim to watch the kids so you can do something for yourself? I'm sure he wouldn't mind."

"Oh, no!" she added quickly. "He's great that way. He watches the kids whenever I have a meeting, and he gets them breakfast on Sunday morning so I can sleep late. That's not the problem."

"What's the problem then?"

"I don't want time to do things by myself. I want time to do things with Jim, but it never happens. He's always doing something. Not for himself, of course — for us: getting the wood ready, refinishing the basement, fixing the car. Important things. He's really a very good husband, you know."

"Yes, I know." There was nothing I could do to help her, but I knew just the person who could. I had worked with her on a case very similar to this, and the results had been quite satisfying.

"I'm going to refer you to someone, Eleanor. I think she can help you solve your problem."

"A therapist? I knew it. I'm neurotic. It's all my fault." She started to cry.

"It's not a therapist. You're not neurotic. And it's definitely not your fault." I wrote the name and telephone number down on a prescription slip and handed it to Eleanor. "Try it. What have you got to lose?"

Eleanor took the paper, put it in her pocketbook, and left.

*   *   *

That evening at Family Report Trine told us, "Eleanor Contremond stopped by to pick up Darlene. We had a nice talk. I really like her. We're going to go out to the mountain to have dinner on Friday, just the two of us. By the way, she said to tell you she thinks everything is going to work out."

I nodded in acknowledgment but was too busy with my mashed potatoes to say anything in response.

After supper, Trine and I were having tea and the kids were playing Go Fish. As she often was when her brood was gathered around her, Trine was in an expansive mood.

"Kids, I want you to know something. Training husbands is a lot of work. Take your father, for example. Here he was, eager to learn and already housebroken when I got him, but it's taken the better part of twelve years to whip him into shape. I want you both to keep that in mind. Especially you, Nadya. Someday you will probably have to do the same thing. You know why? Because husbands are hopeless. Whose fault is it? Mothers'! Mothers who raise their sons to be husbands, so that well-meaning boys like you, Matt, turn out completely ruined. It's a shame. If mothers did the job right, wives wouldn't have to." Nadya and Matt shook their heads in vigorous assent. They had not the foggiest notion what she was talking about, but they knew that it was important for them to show enthusiasm for the lesson.

Later that night, when we were in bed, Trine cuddled up to me. "I'm so lucky I married you," she said, handing me Eleanor's prescription. "You're such a wonderful husband. With a little more training, you might even make a passable wife."

13

*I*t *should have been snowing.* Instead, descending from above was a not-quite-liquid substance that produced, upon striking the body, an invigorating effect not unlike that of bird-shot at five paces. It was a day to sit in a comfortable chair, look out the window, and be thankful you didn't have to go anywhere. The perfect day for a runner to satisfy his debased cravings.

SERIOUS READER NOTE: Among those whose inclination is more toward the sedentary, it is commonly held that the runner is a jogger who has speeded up. This is not true. The distinction between the two is not simply in their method of propulsion. Jogging is an act of locomotion that is distinguished from walking by the fact that both feet may be in the air at the same time, while running requires one to move his legs forward with ever-increasing force and rapidity until he reaches exhaustion. To consider them but two forms of the same activity is akin to saying that, except for the vestments, all religions are identical. There are numerous differences between joggers and runners.

Joggers jog because it makes them feel healthy, because they like to wear bright-colored clothing, and because everybody else does it. The motto of a jogger is "If it feels good, do it."

Runners run because it makes them feel superior, because it hurts, and because they are unable not to. Runners say, "No pain, no gain."

Jogging is a fad.

Running is a disease.

Accordingly, if a person has a friend or family member who has become a jogger, he need not be concerned. The disorder is self-limited. However, if the diagnosis is runner, the prognosis is not nearly so rosy. Distinguishing between the two is not difficult if one looks for the following signs:

Joggers' shoes are always clean.	*Runners' toenails are black.*
Joggers wear gold chains.	*Runners wear watches that calculate lap time, velocity, and blood endorphin levels.*
Joggers smile a lot.	*If you tell a runner you tried running and found it about as much fun as mowing the lawn, he won't laugh.*

———— ◄ ► ————

At the corner of Hill and Maple, I made a right turn and headed toward Stedsville. Three miles after the road changes to dirt, I turned right and entered the woods. Parked just inside the woods, in a small clearing, was a yellow VW bug with California plates. On the rear of the car was a bumper sticker that said "If God Had Wanted People to Have Nuclear Weapons, She Would Have Given Us Lead Skin." A twinge of nostalgia wafted up from hibernation in my temporal lobe and lodged in my frontal cortex, preempting considerations about what pace would be appropriate for these weather conditions. Whose was it? I wondered. I knew of no other West Coast expatriate residing in Dumster. But I did not wonder long. The hill was waiting.

The trail ahead of me ascended gradually for almost a mile until it reached the top of a long ridge. After traversing the ridge, it then veered to the right and descended precipitously into a gully below. Although the grade was not steep, there was enough mud on the ground to give the climb good moral value. I slipped and sloshed my way to the summit. Thirty-five minutes and fifteen seconds. Three twenty-seven slower than my personal record. For these conditions, it was a good time. My T-shirt and shorts were at one with the elements. My knees complained bitterly. Goose bumps rose from my skin like boiling water. I felt good. From here, the trip was all downhill. Fifteen minutes and I would be home. Twenty and I would be in the tub. I carefully picked my way down the rocky path.

At the bottom, a spring-swollen stream bounded through the gully as it made its disheveled descent to Sted Brook. At the junction of the stream and the trail was a young woman. She was kneeling on the ground, and her concentration appeared to be focused on something immediately beneath her. As I got closer, I could see that the object of her interest was a dog.

Bursting with Good Samaritan thoughts, I ran down to her. Eschewing the usual pleasantries that transpire when a man meets a woman in the middle of the woods, she went straight to the point.

"Do you have any peanut butter?"

The substance she requested forms the foundation of my nutritional habitat. As ill luck would have it, however, I was at present without. Disappointed, I confessed my failure. I invited her to the house where, I assured her, the larder was much better stocked.

"Oh, it's not for me. It's for Shira." Seeing the puzzled look on my face, she added, "I'm Sunrise Holbode. We just moved here from California."

We hugged.

"Pleased to meet you. My name is Beach. If I'm not being too inquisitive, perhaps you might explain — "

"About the peanut butter? Shira has hypoglycemia."

"Hypoglycemia? Of course. How foolish of me. It should have been obvious."

"That's what her chiropractor said when I told him about her symptoms. Told me it was a classic case. He recommended peanut butter for treatment of her attacks. Usually I bring it with me wherever we go, but today I left it in the car."

"That's most interesting. I've never heard of hypoglycemia in a dog. What are her symptoms?"

"She can't run uphill. Every time she tries, she breaks into a sweat and falls down. It's pretty bad. Sometimes, just looking at a hill can bring on an attack."

"And just by feeding her peanut butter, you can get her to climb hills?"

"Not always. Sometimes I have to carry her."

I looked at the contented-appearing dog. I looked at her rain-soaked owner. I have treated many cases of hypoglycemia, and I have heard a myriad of its symptoms, but never before had I seen anything like this. Hypoglycemia as a cause of common sense.

SERIOUS READER NOTE: *There is no situation that puts a greater strain on the doctor-patient relationship than one in which the patient complains of a problem for which the doctor can find no excuse. The doctor is then faced with giving one of two equally unpleasant speeches: he can either tell the patient that nothing is wrong, or he can admit that he doesn't have the faintest idea what is going on.*

It might seem, at first blush, that nothing would make a person happier than to hear that her pesky little ache is not a harbinger that her ultimate demise — full broadside and flags flying — will soon be hoving into view. However, when a patient has gone to all the trouble of working herself into a snit about what she considers to be a pretty good set of symptoms, and then she brings them in to her doctor and Sawbones tells her it's nothing but a false alarm . . . well, that can be a pretty stiff blow to the old ego. A patient treated like that may think twice before trundling back in again the next time she's off her feed.

And it isn't any more consoling to hear from Mighty Healer that the symptoms she has submitted for inspection certainly are worthy of attention, and he is glad she came in to report them, but, if she wants to know what he thinks has caused them, well, he doesn't have the foggiest — although it probably isn't anything too awful, because he knows most of the awful ones and it doesn't sound like any of them. Under circumstances like these, a patient might not just become upset; she might lose faith in her doctor. This would not be good. Faith is important to people, and in this day and age, when all our idols cheat or take drugs, it can be pretty hard to come by. It's gotten to the point where the faith market has so dried up that there are only two sources of investment left. If people lose faith in their doctors, all that remains is the lottery.

For this reason, the profession has always had at its disposal a couple of diseases for those symptoms that never quite fit into any diagnostic basket. Back in the good old days, there was a wide variety to choose from. Asthenia. Consumption. Malaria. Dropsy. Today, one label fits all. Dizzies, dumps, or drags. Blahs, bloats, or blues. Claustrophobia, photophobia, or hillophobia. There's room for everything under its big tent. No ache too minor. No ailment too obscure. That's the hypoglycemia creed.

The beauty of hypoglycemia is that it can account for any symptom, as long as that symptom occurs after eating. Since, at any given point in time, there is usually some preceding time at which food was consumed, the potential for symptom justification is limitless.

"I'll carry her. Good workout for the old legs." Brain was quite pleased with this gallant offer. Knees accused Brain of losing its lid.

"Gee, thanks. That would be wonderful. I'd do it myself, but my asthma started acting up. It isn't far. My car is practically around the corner."

Topographically speaking, Sunrise was correct. Unfortunately, the corner in question was the back side of this hill, negotiation of which would require traveling most of the way in the stream. I shouldered Shira and started back up in the direction I had just come from. Sunrise followed right behind me, discoursing on the virtues of real weather, a meteorological phenomenon that she distinguished from the unreal variety by the presence of climatic conditions such as those we were presently experiencing. Listening to Sunrise's mellow babblings, I remembered California weather: always sunny, always warm — weather that made you want to lie down and take a nap. Just a little nap.

Suddenly Sunrise was shouting. At me.

"Beach! Get up!"

Ignoring my protests that I should be allowed to finish

my nap, Sunrise rousted me from my position of repose on the ground. Somehow all three of us got back to the car. While I shivered in the front seat, and Shira relaxed in the back, Sunrise stuffed us both with peanut butter.

"I feel awful," she said. "The doctor never told me it was contagious. If I'd known, I never would have — "

"Hey. It's OK, really. Besides, I think my attack of hypo is more of the thermic variety."

"Oh, no! It's hypoglycemia. Your symptoms are identical to Shira's. You really ought to see a doctor about it."

"That would be awkward, Sunrise. You see, I am a doctor."

"You? No! But you seem so real. Ohmigod! This is incredible. I figured I would never find a doctor out here I could relate to, and now — What are you?"

"Gemini," I said. I was born a Leo, but when I moved to Berkeley I converted. Geminis relate better.

"I can't believe this karma! I'm a Gemini too. And it wouldn't be too much hassle — I mean, you'll really take care of me?"

"I'd love to."

Sunrise Holbode undressed methodically. She folded each article of clothing neatly and placed it on the chair before she proceeded with the next. Shoes. Stockings. Skirt. Blouse. Shivers of excitement ran down my spine as I watched her unwrap her magnificent body. She leaned forward, gracefully arching her willowy spine so that I might unsnap her bra. When she swung around to face me again, she was stark naked. Trembling, I thought I would melt in a pool of molten ecstasy. Intent upon other acts, my lips refused to form the words I wanted to say. I pointed mutely at the bed. Eagerly she climbed up, her long, slender legs extended as she lay there looking at me expectantly. Gently, I parted her smooth thighs. One thought burned in my brain:

It's a good thing doctors aren't perverts.

SERIOUS READER NOTE: Serious readers have no doubt noted a definite change in my literary style. You should disregard the above passage. It has nothing to do with my examination of Sunrise Holbode. It was written at the suggestion of my agent solely to revive the interest of the sex fiends, who, she pointed out, are far more numerous than serious readers.

Professionally speaking, which is the only way I plan to talk on the subject, looking at a naked body should be no big deal. The reproductive and dermatological parts have no more medical interest than the digestive or the circulatory. Unfortunately, not all physicians have learned this. Even the best barrel always has a few rotten apples. And because people place so much faith in us, it is easy to overlook them, for things that would be considered abnormal or even bizarre if an ordinary person did them can be done by doctors with impunity. Like seeing people you hardly know undressed.

SERIOUS READER NOTE: Perversion is an uncommon but serious problem in the medical profession. It is important for all pa-

tients to be on the alert for any signs of deviant tendencies on the part of their physicians. Here are some of them:

1. *The doctor examines you with a warm stethoscope.*
2. *The doctor undresses before asking you to undress.*
3. *The doctor always says you need massage therapy no matter what your complaints are.*
4. *The doctor is on time.*

A doctor's-eye view of the body is actually quite boring. For example, this is what I wrote about Sunrise in her medical record.

S.H. 26yo WDWNWF
Skin: w/o lesions, cyanosis, icterus
HEENT: neg
Chest: clear to P&A
Cor: w/o m, rubs, gallops
Breasts: w/o masses or asymmetry
Abd: w/o organomegaly
Pelvic:
    Introitus: nl
    Cx: w/o erosion
    Uterus: NSSP
    Adnexae: NF
Ext: full ROM w/o pain

Translated, it says that Sunrise was not unduly thin nor excessively fat. Her integument was not discolored and was free of unauthorized protuberances. The air moved through her as silently as the wind. Her hollow organs were empty. Her solid ones, full. The moving parts did so without complaint, and the stationary ones stayed put. Her orifices were clean as a whistle. Hers was, in short, a normal body.

With one exception. Despite the fact that the room was a comfortable Southern California warm, Sunrise was shaking like a leaf.

"Maybe you should put your clothes on," I suggested. "You look cold."

"That's just it. I'm not at all. But I shake all the time. I can hardly hold a teacup."

"How long has this been a problem?"

"Ever since I came out East. I assumed it was just a yin imbalance from the move, so I didn't think anything of it, but I've been here almost a month and it's no better."

"Yin could certainly be the culprit, especially the yin from your asthma medicine."

"I don't take any. It keeps me from hearing what my body is saying to me. And my asthma: it hasn't bothered me at all since I came here. Usually it acts up whenever I'm in a new place."

"That is strange. Do you drink much coffee or tea? Sometimes caffeine can cause a reaction like this."

"I know. One cup of coffee and I'll twitch like a jitterbug. All I take is chamomile. That shouldn't cause any problems, should it?"

"No. Any new supplements or tonics? You can find stimulants in the strangest places sometimes."

"Nothing — except guarana, but that couldn't do anything. It's organic."

"Guarana? Isn't that another word for bat dung?"

"No, silly." She laughed. "That's guano. Guarana is a natural energizer from South America. It's great stuff. I ordered it from my *Whole Mother Earth Catalog*. They recommended it for adjusting to new environments."

"Hmmm. Never heard of it. Do you have the bottle with you?"

"Yup. It's right here." She pulled a small brown bottle from her pocket and handed it to me. I read the label.

GUARANA

Share the secret of the Amazon women. This amazing South American wonder herb lifts spirits and lowers appetite. Cures headaches, depression, and asthma with nature's own healing energy. Revel at your body and watch others do the same. Drug free. Completely organic. Guaranteed results.

"Do you mind if I show this to one of my partners? He knows a lot more about this kind of stuff than I do." Sunrise thought that would be fine, so I went over to Dale Hurbalife's office. Dr. Hurbalife was our resident expert in matters floral.

"Very interesting," he said. "I've never seen this in a pill. This stuff must pack quite a wallop."

"What's in it?"

"Guarana is an extract from the seed of a Brazilian shrub, *Paullinia sorbilis*. After the coca leaf, it's probably the most potent stimulant in the botanical world. It is named after the Guarani Indians, whose warlike behavior is attributed to their consumption of a beverage made from an extract of the leaves. The Guarani are apparently so fierce that if they didn't all die from heart trouble shortly after reaching adulthood, the tribe would probably have conquered all of South America. What you've got here is pure caffeine. I would guess one of these pills has the pharmacological equivalent of three cups of coffee."

I went back and relayed this information to Sunrise. She was aghast.

"But how can anything that's organic be a drug? It doesn't seem possible."

"You wouldn't think anything was safer than air, would you? But too much oxygen can blind a newborn baby and kill an old man with emphysema. Too much water will put you in a coma. Too much vitamin A ruins your liver. Too much vitamin D shuts off your kidneys. Taken to excess, even the most natural substances can be deadly poisons. Nothing is absolutely safe."

"Gosh, Beach. If I can't trust *Whole Mother Earth,* who can I trust?"

"Me, Sunrise."

14

Everyone agreed that Delbert Snide would take over Snide Enterprises when his brother died. (Retirement was not an option for Clarence, whose sole purpose in life was acquisition.) Delbert was in charge of the flagship family business, Snide's Laundromat. He ran it with an iron hand and a tight fist that left no doubt about whether he deserved his position as heir apparent.

When we first moved into our house, it was not yet equipped with a washer and dryer. Since my line of travel took me closer to the Laundromat, I was given responsibility for taking care of the laundry. I was appointed to this post with no little trepidation on Trine's part, for laundry is one of the few aspects of our life where our philosophies differ. I am a one-for-all-and-all-in-one egalitarian, while Trine believes devoutly in a strict class system: reds and blues forever separate, and woe to the T-shirt who tries to mingle with nylons. But when it came right down to it, and she had to make a choice between principle and convenience, even Trine yielded to the demands of the flesh.

Snide's Laundromat is one of Dumster's popular entertainment spots — for women, at least. Men seemed to prefer the environs of Nat's Lunch and the Legion Hall. Maybe this was why I never quite got the hang of watching clothes slosh back and forth or the laundry-fold-and-gossip combo. Accordingly, it was my custom to put the clothes in the washer, return to the hospital, come back to put them in the dryer, and then repeat the sequence to retrieve the clothes from the dryer. Sometimes I got a little delayed and didn't make it back in time to empty the machine, but the women who frequented the Laundromat were so touched to see a doctor doing laundry that one of them would set the clothes aside for me. Delbert was less sentimental than his patrons. He considered my behavior a flagrant abuse of Laundromat policy, which was boldly stated on a large sign above the washers:

LEAVE IT?

LOST IT!

One particularly hectic morning I forgot about my laundry completely. By the time I remembered, it was late afternoon. No one was in the Laundromat except Delbert. I went to the washer to retrieve my clothes. They were gone. I inspected the dryers. Empty. I asked Delbert if he had found a pile of unclaimed laundry. Delbert shrugged and pointed to the sign.

I was looking forward to meeting Delbert again.

SERIOUS READER NOTE: Among the multitude of life's labors, one type has been singled out for special recognition: the professions. The professions are generally acknowledged to be more meritorious endeavors, and those who engage in work so classified are accorded similar esteem. Of the many characteristics that distinguish a profession from ordinary work and that justify one's charg-

*ing an outrageous fee for one's services, by far the most important
is professionalism. Professionalism is the ability to keep your personal feelings from interfering with doing your job. While it is
perfectly acceptable for a secretary to kick the typewriter when a
letter jams, or a plumber to give the old heave-ho to a wrench when
two pipes don't meet quite as they should, a baseball player who
flings his bat after striking out is out of line. And a doctor who takes
out his frustrations on a patient is most definitely not playing
according to Hoyle. In the good old days this was never a problem.
Doctors could always rely on their nurses and wives to absorb the
excess tension that builds up in the course of a normal day of saving
lives. No more. Should I try to relax at home with a little sulking,
Trine would kick me out of the house. And the other day, when I
was a little snappy in flaunting my authority, Sarah actually told
me to shut up. This means that I have no choice other than to pick
on my patients.*

━━━━━━━◄ ♦ ►━━━━━━━

It was the end of a bad week when Delbert Snide came
in to see me. For three days running, I had been up most
of the night with a very sick patient. I had tried every
trick in my bag in a mostly futile effort to get rid of his
fever and abdominal pain. I had stuck tubes into every
cavity I could find, sucked out whatever fluids were contained therein, and replaced them with enough of my
own choosing that even the most recalcitrant case of
diverticulitis — the illness in question — should have cried
uncle. But it hadn't. I discovered why on Thursday when
I consulted Carl Cutterup. He said, "You can feed a pig
birdseed, but it won't make him fly." And then he took
him into the operating room to repair his leaking abdominal aortic aneurysm. Through no fault of mine, the patient pulled through. I had made a bad mistake, and I felt

awful. I had violated a basic rule of medicine: when the patient doesn't respond, consider a new diagnosis before trying a new treatment.

Trine was furious. Each night I had called up to say, "Put supper on the table. I'm just about to leave," only to show up about two hours later. And to top it all off, I hadn't even had time to have tea with Sarah. So I was ready for Delbert.

Delbert Snide looked about as comfortable in a doctor's office as a camel on a flying trapeze. Instead of sitting in the chair, he crouched in the far corner of the room, trying, I assumed, to put as much distance as possible between the two of us by so doing. His coarse features were accentuated by a look of suppressed insolence on his acne-scarred face. When he saw me, his nostrils flared and his lips curled up like the prow of a ship, presenting the two tobacco-stained hulks that were all that remained of its original cargo. Resembling more an animal trapped in a cage than a patient waiting to be examined, he did not appear enthralled with the impending rematch.

"Nice to see you again, Mr. Snide," I greeted him from a safe distance. "What can I do for you?"

"I'm sick," he snarled.

"I'm sorry to hear that. Perhaps you could give me a hint as to the nature of your sickness."

"Won't eat. Don't sleep. Can't work. Got the sweats, the shakes, and the trots. Can't sit still. Can't lie down. I ain't worth *shit!*"

This response, delivered in slightly under fifteen seconds, had obviously been prepared beforehand. There was no point in asking him any further questions. Delbert Snide had told me all he was going to. No matter. The symptoms he had offered were not ready to be assigned a diagnosis and treatment. They needed a bit more time.

SERIOUS READER NOTE: An illness is like an apple: it should be allowed to ripen fully before it is picked from the tree. The physician who attempts to sample his fruit prematurely will find that it is highly inedible. Although the judicious use of tests and pills may hasten its maturation, this is no substitute for a healthy dose of tincture of time. Consequently, the prudent doctor will not hasten to a conclusion about a patient's symptoms upon his first visit, but will have him return after a suitable interval for reexamination, at which time his problem may be more amenable to a definitive diagnosis. However, the doctor must be careful not to wait too long, for if the fruit becomes overripe, it will fall from the tree and rot on the ground, thus denying the physician his just desert.

"Indeed, I believe. Yes. Definitely, indeed. And very interesting. I think we can safely say that something is wrong. It could be a bug. Then again, it couldn't. It may be something. Or it may be something else."

Delbert's face was blank. If he was frightened, he certainly wasn't letting on.

"We'll need some tests, of course — a blood count and urinalysis at least, and perhaps a sample of your stool. We'll make a return appointment for three weeks. In the meantime, take these pills twice a day."

I gave him his prescription and started to get up from my desk. Delbert sprang for the door and was through it before I had reached my feet.

When Delbert Snide came back for his follow-up visit, he was a changed man. His hair was combed, his fingernails were trimmed, and his clothes were clean. He even had a new set of teeth. I couldn't believe the transformation before my eyes. What had happened? Was it the pills? It was hard to believe a few valium could do this much to a man. Maybe I was starting to get a little of the Old Doc Franklin touch.

"You're looking much better today, Mr. Snide. How are you feeling?"

"Mean as the wart on a witch's tit," he snarled. Apparently his transformation had not been complete.

All his tests had turned up nothing. Likewise his physical examination. I was puzzled. I had certainly waited long enough for the problem either to declare itself or to go away, but it had done neither. Yet something was rotten in the state of Delbert, there could be no doubt on that score. Could he be depressed? Even my limited exposure to the Snides had been enough to convince me that they were congenitally immune to disorders of the human spirit, but medicine is a Pandora's box of surprises. There was no harm in asking.

"Are you unhappy, Delbert?"

"Hell, no!"

I could remove depression from diagnostic consideration. I was at a loss as to what to do next. Ordinarily, I would order some more tests and try out another brand of pills, but I was pretty sure that Delbert considered his abbreviated performance as Patient to have been much too long already. For want of any better ideas, I tried honesty.

"I don't know what's going on, Delbert. Everything checks out OK."

"Sumpin's wrong." He was not going to let me off the hook that easily.

I looked at Delbert closely. He looked good. Better, in fact, than I had ever seen him. That was it! He looked *too* good. What a fool I had been! Had Delbert been a seventeen-year-old schoolboy, I would have made the diagnosis immediately. I had never seen a case in an old man, but there could be no doubt. Delbert Snide was in an ARP.

SERIOUS READER NOTE: Acute Romantic Phase, ARP for short, is one of the romance disorders. Its somatic manifestations, although numerous, are of minor importance. Not so its effects on the central nervous system. The patient with delirium arpens is agitated and euphoric. His judgment is markedly impaired, and he is prone to impulsive actions. Unless promptly treated, serious complications can result.

"You are in love," I told him.

Delbert blushed. At least he acted as if he were blushing. On his face, it was impossible to tell. "How'd you know?"

"That doesn't matter. What's important is to find out how serious it is."

Delbert studied his shoes carefully. "We was thinking of getting hitched."

"Don't."

"Don't get hitched?"

"Don't think. It's too dangerous. Tell me this: have you been married before?"

Delbert consulted his shoes again. "Once."

"For how long?"

"Two years."

"That's not long enough."

"If you'da knowed her, you wouldn't say that."

"That's not what I mean. Two years isn't long enough for

a training marriage to confer protection against the complications of your condition. How long have you felt like this?"

"She been coming to the Laundromat 'bout six months. A real lady, she is. Always takes her laundry out right on time. Not like some people. I didn't pay her much mind until 'bout two months ago. Her machine broke, and I had to go fix it. You know how it is with them washing machines. One thing led to another, and pretty soon she was bringing in her laundry every day."

Delbert's voice softened as he talked about his new love. He looked relaxed. And on his lips was the slight hint of a smile. There was no mistaking it. Delbert Snide was in full ARP. He was too old for the traditional treatment, emotional guardianship by a responsible adult. There was only one course of action possible.

"Move in with her."

He recoiled as if I had struck him. "I couldn't do that. Besides she'd never agree."

"There is no alternative. Consider it as a lease–purchase option for your marriage. By the way, who is the lucky woman?"

"Ann Waters."

I took out my prescription pad and wrote — legibly, for it was not going to a pharmacist —

Delbert Snide

For medical reasons,
This patient must, until further notice,
Reside with Ms. Ann Waters

Beach Conger, M.D.

Delbert looked at the prescription. "How long?"
"Until the ARP is over."

"How can I tell?"

"There are many ways. The most reliable is the automobile stress test. The first time you tell her not to drive so fast, and she tells you to mind your own business, the ARP is gone. Then you can get married . . . if you still want to."

⅔ *15* ⅃

President for Life of the Stedsville Historical Society, Chairperson of Friends of Stedsville Cemetery, Founder of the Stedsville Polo Club — these were but a smattering of her list of contributions to the Stedsville community. Despite an impressive collection of distinguished citizens — which includes, in addition to Henry Turnstill, a former Supreme Court justice, two famous authors, and a movie star — Buffy Uprite reigns supreme as undisputed monarch of Stedsville. Buffy and her late husband, Alexander Cabot Uprite III, came to Stedsville in 1965, bringing with them as much of Buffy's inheritance and Alexander's lineage as the move would permit, which was considerably more of the former than the latter. They purchased four hundred acres of outer Stedsville's most scenic countryside property with the intention of using it as the summer component of their domestic complement, the other elements of which were a house in Grand Cayman Island and a pied-à-terre on Beacon Hill. Alex tolerated the bucolic environment surprisingly well for a man of his upbringing, although not for periods of more than a week at a time, and even then not without daily calls to his man in Boston. The stated purpose of these calls was to check on "the state of

things," which, befitting a man of his stature, were undoubt-
edly numerous and in need of close supervision. Buffy had
no such need. She was captivated by the quiet charm of
rural living, and she was quite content to declare that the
one-story glass-and-steel wraparound they had built into
the southwestern slope of Goreham Hill was their home.

Buffy is a woman of action. There is hardly an aspect of
life into which she has not plunged with boundless energy.
She has mobilized. She has organized. She has actualized.
Her life experience has been, in a word, full. But though
she is a woman of many pleasures, Buffy Uprite has only
one love. To the particular dismay of neither of them, this
love is not and was never her once dear, now departed Alex.
Buffy loves horses. She has a stable of Arabians that is
considered, by those who profess to know about such things,
to be one of the finest collections of horseflesh in the country. An accomplished equestrienne, she spends most of her
time either riding her horse trails or worshipping at the
temple she has erected to commemorate her love: the Stedsville Polo Field.

The road from downtown Stedsville to Buffy's winds for
several miles through a maze of thick pines. Just before it
reaches the farm, the road makes a sharp right turn, at
which point the woods end abruptly and the polo field
springs into view. Even though I have seen it many times, it
never fails to take my breath away. To an eye whose vision
has been accustomed to the dark and cozy woods, this huge
expanse of perfectly flat, manicured light-green lawn is like
. . . it's like this: if God decided to take up golf, Buffy
Uprite's polo field would be his putting green.

Buffy is a friendly soul. A person meeting her for the first
time, unaware of her social position, would think she was
just an ordinary person — unless, of course, he happened
to suggest to Buffy that she might do something that did
not suit her, and then he would quickly be disabused of his

illusion. Buffy is accustomed to having her own way. She has that graceful arrogance of the established rich that is handed down in a family from generation to generation like an ancient heirloom. Elegant yet not obtrusive, Buffy's arrogance fits her as if it were tailor-made. Had she so chosen, Buffy would have made a fine doctor.

There is one trouble with a life like Buffy's. Never having included a skirmish with adversity, it leaves a person ill prepared to deal with the inevitable vicissitudes that pop up as one approaches the end of her shuffle along the mortal coil. Buffy Uprite has never, in all of her fifty-five years, even considered the possibility that her existence might someday contain an obstacle that she could not, through the force of influence, easily hurdle. Whether getting a polo field built in the rocky hills of Vermont or putting an end to the nuclear arms race, Buffy is sure that solving any problem is simply a matter of getting in touch with the Right People.

Two weeks ago, Buffy came in to correct some swelling in her hands.

"Beach, darling. Terribly sorry to bother you. It's so silly, really. You must have so many more important things to do with all those awfully sick patients of yours, poor things. I don't know how they put up with it. It's these hands. I just can't get them to behave. Every time it gets cold, they puff up like balloons. And they ache so, I could simply scream. They're utterly hopeless. It's such a bore. Here, look at them." She briefly waved the offending parts in front of me and then returned them to the safety of her lap. "Be a good dear and fix them for me."

SERIOUS READER NOTE: Before any readers become too upset at Buffy's apparent indiscretion, I should hasten to point out that there

are two circumstances under which it is acceptable to address a
doctor by his first name:

    *1. If there is an emergency, e.g., "Beach, your pants are
      on fire."*
    2. If you are rich.

    I examined Buffy's hands. Her finger joints were swollen,
red, and warm to the touch.

    "Osteoarthritis. A mild case. Three aspirin four times a
day for a couple of weeks should take care of the acute
inflammation."

    "Aspirin?" Buffy arched her voice slightly at my mention
of the drug.

    "On the other hand," I replied, correcting my error, "you
might do better with Feldene. It's an excellent drug."

    Feldene is the newest of the nonsteroidal anti-
inflammatory drugs. It is a fine pill. Each one costs over a
dollar.

---

*SERIOUS READER NOTE: Nonsteroidal anti-inflammatory
drugs, NSAIDs for short, have revolutionized the treatment of arthritis. Prior to NSAIDs, when people with arthritis came to see the
doctor, all he could say was take two aspirin and come back next year.
They usually didn't bother to come back. A few became so disillusioned
with health care that they dropped out of the system altogether. But
most of them defected to chiropractors. With the advent of NSAIDs
(which are virtually identical to aspirin except for being a little*

*easier on the stomach and a little harder on the kidneys), they
returned to the fold eager to try out the wonder drugs.*

*Several years ago, ibuprofen, generic name for Motrin, the first
of the NSAIDs, became available over the counter. Fears that this
would cut into the arthritis trade quickly disappeared when it turned
out that the drug would only be marketed in two-hundred-milligram
tablets. Side by side, a puny Advil and the eight-hundred-
milligram, still-prescription-only Super Motrin look like a Carter's
Little Liver Pill and an MX missile. Anyway, by the time it went on
the shelves, Motrin had become as obsolete in the NSAID market as
last year's designer jeans.*

"Thanks ever so," Buffy bubbled, taking her prescription. "I feel cured already. You and Trine really ought to
stop by for a drink sometime. It would be nice to see you
outside the office for a change."

It was a typical Buffy Uprite gesture. Friendly, generous,
and not at all intended to be taken seriously.

"We'd love to."

Eleven-thirty on Saturday night, the phone rang, awak-
ening me from a sound sleep. It was Buffy.

"Beach, dear? Thank goodness it's you. I'd hate to get a
wrong number at this hour. Terribly sorry to bother you,
but — you're not asleep, are you?"

"Heavens, no! Trine and I were just sitting around the
fire discussing how to redecorate our living room." Years of
experience had taught me how to answer virtually any question promptly and plausibly without being fully awake.

"Marvelous. Well, you know those darling little pills you
gave me? The pretty blue ones?"

"Feldene."

"Yes. That's it. Well, I hate to say it, dear, but I'm afraid they didn't work."

"Impossible!"

"It's true. For the first few days, everything was fine. But tonight I tried to pick up my teacup, and I couldn't get my finger through the handle. I had to hold it like a mug. It was dreadful."

"Sounds pretty serious. I'll be right over."

"That would be sweet. You're sure it isn't too much of a bother?"

"Not at all. I was just thinking of going out for a midnight ski. It helps me get to sleep."

"Thanks ever so. See you in a jiff."

I rummaged through my dresser for a pair of knickers and wool socks with which to make good my lie. Trine, aroused by my fumblings, to the likes of which she had long since become immune, stirred in the bed. "Emergency?" she mumbled sleepily.

"No. Buffy!"

"Oh." She turned over and fell asleep again. Ordinarily Trine was quite outraged on my behalf if a patient dared to call me at home. Buffy, however, allowed us to ski on her horse trails and use her heated swimming pool. There are few things Trine loves more than good skiing and warm water. I am allowed to pamper Buffy without fear of reproach.

When I got to the house, Buffy was holding a dinner party. "This is my doctor, Beach." She introduced me to the assembled guests much as she might one of her prized equestrian possessions. "He's such a dear. I don't know what I would do without him." She offered me a drink, which I refused, and then her hands, which I accepted.

They were considerably improved since last I had had the privilege of inspecting them. The swelling was greatly diminished, and though the telltale Heberden's nodes were still there, that was to be expected. They always would be.

"Are they very painful?" I asked, somewhat mystified by the cause for her concern. Buffy had a pretty high tolerance for pain, and it was hard to believe that the digits I had just seen could create any significant discomfort.

"Heavens, no! The pain is all gone. But look at them. They're so ugly." She flourished the miscreants before her guests, who murmured in assent.

"I'm afraid they're always going to look like that, Buffy. Medication will lessen the symptoms of arthritis, but it can't do anything to stop the disease itself. Of course, you could have the joints replaced." I added this last observation solely with the intent of preempting any such suggestion on her part. "But I wouldn't recommend it."

"I'm sure you're right," said Buffy, the temperature in her voice dropping about twenty degrees as she turned to her guests. "There's nobody like my Beach. Beach went to Harvard." She offered this observation not so much to prove her statement — proof being a commodity for which Buffy had never had use — but because her description of me would not be complete without mention of my pedigree.

"What is your specialty, young man?" asked one of the guests, who seemed singularly unimpressed with my appearance.

"I'm an internist."

"Ah. An internist. Internist." His mouth puckered slightly as he repeated the word, as if it had a sour taste to it.

"Arthur is very interested in arthritis," explained Buffy. "He is president of the Massachusetts Society for the Preservation of Joints, and his grandfather built that darling little hospital up on Parker Hill. You know, the one with such a lovely view of Brookline?"

I knew. I had lived beneath it for four years. It is the foremost arthritis center in the country.

"Arthur was telling me about this marvelous doctor down there — a hand man — who's simply done wonders for everyone. Arthur — he's such a dear — thought that he might be able to help me . . . if you agree, of course."

"Would you like me to call him now?" I suspected that the Boston specialist was not accustomed to be awakened at midnight for routine appointments, but I was never quite sure where the limits of propriety lay for those in Buffy's class.

"That won't be necessary. I wouldn't want to bother him at this hour. Why don't you give him a ring sometime tomorrow?"

"I'll do it first thing in the morning."

Buffy thanked me profusely. Arthur gave me the rheumatologist's card, and I made my exit.

One of the nicest aspects of practicing in Dumster is that most patients trust my judgment. Should I happen to recommend a second opinion, they would be perfectly agreeable. But they would be no more likely to suggest it on their own than they would to Ben Smith on a difficult hardware case or Cliff Bender down at Dumster Texaco for a complicated automotive problem. Patients like this make a doctor feel competent and useful. Then there are patients like Buffy, who listen politely to my opinion but, no matter how brilliant my pronouncement on the affliction in point, invariably suggest that perhaps it might be wise to consult a specialist before doing anything too precipitously. Patients who make me feel like a dope.

––––––◄ ♦ ►––––––

Serious reader note: Internists have not always been the victims of such shabby treatment. Time was, we were the kings of the medical mountain. Diagnosticians, they called us. It was our job to tell patients what was going on. If a person wanted to be sure there was a proper name for her illness, she went to an internist. That the particular name given to the ailment bore little more than a random relationship to its etiology was unimportant. In those days the treatment of an illness had nothing to do with its cause.

However, once sophisticated laboratory tests enabled us to pinpoint even the most minuscule obscuropathy, the art of disease naming became obsolete, and the internist yielded his throne to an upstart: the specialist. Possessed with prodigious reproductive ability, specialists begat specialists, and the begotten begat subspecialists. Soon there was not a single problem that didn't have a specialist uniquely qualified to treat it. What has that left for the internist? Equipped with no particular skills and possessed of no exalted titles, we ply our trade on the humble and the meek. We are the wimp doctors.

I was tired of being pushed around by this gang of fancy names. I was as good as they were. And I was going to prove it.

First thing Monday morning, I went to the library and got out the AMA Directory of Medical Specialties. I didn't want anything fancy; just a modest little something to gain me a modicum of respect. A something that wouldn't have too much competition. There were a thousand pages and more of specialties, from arthroscopist to zenbuddologist, every one chock-full of doctors. It was pretty discouraging. Then I had an inspiration. The road untraveled. A specialty all to myself. One of my own creation. Imagine! Me, the only specialist of my kind in the entire world. All I had to do was figure out what it would be. The rest would be easy. At Family Report that night, I announced my intentions.

"I've decided to become a specialist."

"What kind?" asked Trine.

"A very exclusive one."

"And where are you planning to pursue this noble endeavor?"

"Washington, D.C."

"Wonderful! What will happen to us, while you engage in this orgy of self-indulgence?"

"I was hoping you might come with me."

"Great. I'll quit school, ship Nadya to Norway, and send Matt back to California, just so I can trundle after you to the Big City."

"Actually, I thought you might enjoy it. It wouldn't be long."

"Let's see. If I remember correctly, in Vermont, 'not long' is a unit of time lasting somewhere between five minutes and five years, as distinguished from 'a long time,' the duration of which covers ten minutes to a lifetime. Perhaps you could convert your estimate into something your poor Flatlander wife could understand?"

"Two days should do it. I was thinking of next weekend. The cherry blossoms should be in full bloom. We'll dump the kids at Eleanor's on Thursday and get a sleeper on Amtrak. That will bring us into D.C. before noon. While I complete my studies, you can watch the Supreme Court in action. Saturday we can do the town, hop on the night train, and we're back home Sunday afternoon. Of course, if you'd rather stay home . . ."

"You sneak!" exclaimed Trine in mock outrage. "I'll get the tickets tomorrow. You handle the child care."

No sooner had we checked into our hotel Friday morning than I headed off to the Library of Congress. The Library of Congress is no ordinary library. It took me the better part of two hours just to find the right building. Once there,

I spent the rest of the day filling out an application for a library card, which required in addition to the usual stuff a complete set of fingerprints and letters of reference from all the libraries I had used in the last ten years. The librarian explained to me that it would take six weeks to process. When I told him I would only be in Washington for two days, he explained that he was just carrying out the intent of Congress. By the time I got back to the hotel, I was pretty depressed.

"Call Leahy," said Trine when I told her what had happened.

"You don't go to your senator to get a library card."

"In America you do."

So first thing Saturday morning I paid a visit to the office of Senator Patrick Leahy. The secretary, who turned out to be a distant relative of Ernest Bouchard, was very helpful. She told me that Senator Leahy would be most pleased to know I had visited, which she would be sure to tell him as soon as he returned from a fact-finding trip to the Fiji Islands — something to do with aid to their dairy farmers. I told her about my troubles at the Library of Congress.

"Heavens," she said, "you should have come here yesterday." She made a quick phone call, and thirty minutes later I was standing in front of the librarian, card in hand. I wondered to him if the intent of Congress had created both the local and express routes to a library card.

"What books would you like?" he replied.

I gave him the list. After a little while, he returned with a large pile of books.

"Funny thing," he said. "I've been here twenty-eight years, and I have never seen anybody interested in this subject. But you're the second one this week. Curious, I'd say."

"Isn't it, though. I suppose he didn't happen to mention what aspect of the field he was interested in," I inquired with what I hoped would pass for an air of professional curiosity.

"Composition. Mentioned something about trying to synthesize it. She was a chemist, I believe."

What a relief! A chemist was no competitor. Who knows, we might even be able to collaborate. I jotted down her name from the checkout card for future reference.

It was a long day, but at the end, my education was complete. No longer one of the masses, I had become a specialist. On the way home, lulled by the gentle rocking of the car and the clackity-clack of the wheels, visions of my new shingle danced in my head.

Beach Conger, M.D.
CERUMENOLOGIST

SERIOUS READER NOTE: For anyone interested in becoming a cerumenologist, I have included in this diary a brief primer of clinical cerumenology. Although it is enough to give one a feeling for the specialty, it is not nearly adequate to equip him to enter into the practice thereof. Those who are serious about it can write to me, and I will be glad to discuss it further.

1. *Earwax is produced by glands in the ear canal in order to protect and lubricate the skin in the canal. It is removed by propulsion from the back-and-forth movement of the jaw, as with eating and talking. There is considerable controversy regarding the fate of earwax once it gets to the end of the canal. Whether it is reabsorbed or simply evaporates into the air is unknown.*

2. *There are two varieties of earwax: wet and dry.*

3. *Some people suffer from a deficiency of earwax. They can be treated with cerumen transplants, a delicate operation that should only be performed by a cerumenologist. There is hope that someday artificial cerumen will obviate the need for such surgery.*

4. *Earwax has a high protein content, but it is also very rich in cholesterol. It should not be eaten.*

5. *Earwax is your friend. Leave it alone. If the Lord had wanted us to remove earwax, he wouldn't have put it where it is.*

⤙ *16* ⤚

*H*er name was Marjorie Dunham, but everyone knew her as Merry. The Dunhams were a distinguished Dumster family. Ever since 1806, when James William Dunham became town agent, there has always been at least one Dunham serving Dumster in a position of public responsibility. Merry had kept the tradition alive by teaching history at Dumster High School for forty-six of her seventy-five years and by remaining a spinster for all seventy-five of them. She was born in the small red house that William had built next to the town hall and had never lived anywhere else. "I'll die in that house," she often said, "and then you can burn both of us."

Merry was the kind of person that makes other people feel good about themselves just because they know her. If a good cause was in need, it was Merry who organized the committee. When someone suffered a personal tragedy, Merry's casserole was first on the doorstep. Her pockets were never without candy for kids, and her mouth was never without a kind word for adults.

Merry came to see me in November about a sore throat.

"I know how busy you are, Dr. Conger. And I hate to bother you with something as silly as a sore throat, but it

keeps me up at night so. Behind the right tonsil, I think.
Well, not exactly behind the tonsil, because Old Doc
Walter — He was before your time. Now there was a won-
derful man. Never thought of himself. Died of consump-
tion, you know; got it from one of his patients. Ellie
Johnson, it was. Little slip of a thing. But pretty as a picture.
Doc Walter tended her every day, and not a few nights too.
She recovered completely — went to New York City and
became a ballet dancer at Radio City Music Hall. But Old
Doc Walter up and died just after she left. Some said that
he — well, you know how people talk, even about doctors.
It's a shame. Anyway, he took out my tonsils. So what I
mean is, the soreness is right where the tonsil used to be."
Without breaking conversational stride, she pointed to the
area in question. "I thought maybe you could give me a little
something to soothe it. That wonderful medicine Doc
Franklin's wife made. Not that I'm trying to tell you how to
do your job. You're the doctor. But I thought I ought to
give you all the information I had — to help you out. I
always say knowledge is like love: you can never get too
much of it."

Merry believed in two things. Knowledge was one; the
other was that it is better to give than to receive. Nothing
pleased her more than to use them both.

"Let's take a look," I said, hoping to kill two birds with
one stone.

She opened her mouth. The throat was a little red but,
given its constant exposure to the elements, no more than I
would have expected. Just to be thorough, I peeked in her
ears, examined her neck, and thumped on her chest. Then
I suggested a chest X ray.

"It's cancer, isn't it?" Merry said matter-of-factly.

I started. "What makes you think that?"

"The look on your face when you were poking around in
my neck. There was something there you didn't like at all.

And when you asked me to get an X ray without discussing the sore throat . . . well, Dr. Conger, it's not like you to be that quiet. You know, sometimes you can tell more about what people are thinking by what they don't say than you can by what they do. Just tell me straight out what you think. You don't have to be afraid."

"Well," I hemmed, "I wouldn't say that I can definitely call it cancer." I hawed, "It could be something else."

"Such as?"

"A condition maybe. Perhaps an inflammation. Could even be a growth, I suppose."

"But what do you think it is?"

She had me. "I think it's cancer."

"Cancer. C-A-N-C-E-R. Greek word. It means crab. Hera (she was Zeus' wife — his twin sister too) named one of the constellations Cancer in honor of the crab who tried to kill Hercules while Hercules was chopping heads off the Lernaen Hydra. Euripedes said there were a thousand, but he exaggerated. There were only seven. Hera hated Hercules. Zeus disguised himself as a mortal once so he could seduce Alcmene. Then Alcmene got pregnant and had Hercules, and Zeus decided to make him a god. But that wasn't the worst of it. Alcmene was out walking with baby Hercules one day, and she met Hera coming in the other direction. Alcmene pretended it was a big surprise, but she had planned it all along. Hera, not knowing that this was her husband-brother's kid, stopped and said, 'What a cute baby.' And Alcmene said, 'Would you like to hold him?' Hera said she would. Well, Hercules grabbed on to her tit and sucked so hard that she jerked away. Milk came shooting out like a volcano, which was how the Milky Way was formed. Hera was hopping mad. Zeus said he would thunderbolt Hera if she messed with Alcmene, so instead she cast a spell on Hercules — not that he had done anything wrong except be born, but that's the way gods were. As long as they got their revenge, they didn't care who was hurt. Hercules, who was grown up by now, went bonkers and killed six of his children, which is pretty horrible, but he had fifty, so by godly standards it wasn't such a big deal. After Hercules recovered, he went into a funk. Zeus talked to him. 'Son,' he said, 'gods don't have funks. I'm going to send you to work for Erytheseus. If you do a good job, immortality is yours. Otherwise, it's off with your head.' Zeus didn't know it, but Erytheseus was in cahoots with Hera. He gave Hercules the hardest job he could think of. Killing the Hydra was the second one. It was while Hercules was fighting the Hydra that the crab came up and bit him on the toe. Hercules was furious. You know what he did?"

Greek mythology was not heavily emphasized in medical education. I so indicated with a silent response. It was a brief silence.

"He stepped on it. This was no ordinary crab, mind you. It was twelve feet across. But Hercules squashed it like a bug. Then, he polished off the Hydra. I wonder what would have happened if we had called it 'crab' instead. Maybe people wouldn't be so afraid. My, how I'm carrying on. Where were we? Oh, yes! Off to X ray it is."

She brought back her film. It showed a big snowball in the left lung.

Merry was unimpressed. "I suppose I'll die."

"Not necessarily," I replied, trying to cushion the shock.

"According to the First Book of Moses, Methuselah lived for nine hundred and sixty-nine years. But it probably wasn't really that long, because back then, they didn't use the Gregorian calendar. I mean, he didn't have his first kid until he was one hundred and eighty-seven, so we have no idea how long a year was. The oldest known human — documented, that is: there are people living in the Caucasus mountains who claim to be over one hundred and fifty years old, but they don't have birth certificates — was Shigechiyo Izumi. He lived for one hundred and twenty years, two hundred and thirty-seven days. He died February twenty-first this year. They asked him once to what he attributed his longevity. 'Two things,' he said. 'Buddha and television.' People are like that. I had an aunt who was convinced that as long as she brushed her hair fifty strokes every morning and chewed every bite of food twenty-five times — or maybe it was twenty-five strokes and fifty chews — she would never get old. Morarji Desai, the former prime minister of India, claims he keeps young by drinking a cup of his own urine each morning. So I suppose anything is possible. Still, I don't understand how getting lung cancer will give me immortality."

"What I meant was that you might not die from the cancer. There's always a chance of cure from surgery. And at your age the cancer might grow slowly enough that you could outlive it."

"You mean I might drop dead from a heart attack or fall down, break my hip, and get a blood clot to the lungs before the cancer gets me? That's good to know. But supposing nothing else carries me off, how long can this cancer and I hang around with each other?"

"That's hard to say. The prognosis for survival varies considerably, depending on the extent and type of tumor."

"I'm not trying to be difficult, Dr. Conger, but I need to know. I'm in charge of the Town Meeting Day Cleanup Drive. If I'm not going to be around then, I ought to resign."

"You won't die before Town Meeting," I said, "from the cancer."

"How about Old Home Day? I'm supposed to lead the parade this year."

"Well . . ."

"So I've got a guarantee until March, but not July. That's

not too bad. There's one other thing I've got to know. Sorry to be such a pest, but it's important. Is it going to hurt? I can't stand pain. It's the only thing I'm afraid of."

"We should be able to control your pain with narcotics, but it takes a little trial and error to find the right dose. I wouldn't want you to get too sedated."

"With all respect, Dr. Conger, if I start hurting, I won't care about being too sedated. If I have to be doped up to be comfortable, then that's what I want. I don't mind dying, but I don't want to suffer."

"I'll do what I can, Merry. You must understand that there are certain ethical considerations regarding care of terminal patients which a physician must consider in administering potentially life-threatening drugs."

"Heavens!" she exclaimed, crestfallen. "I wouldn't want you to do something unethical." She paused for a second. The light in her face switched on again. "How about this? Suppose I ask you to give me a prescription for sleeping pills because I have trouble sleeping. Would you be willing to do that?"

"Of course, relieving suffering is the most important responsibility of a physician."

"Even if I told you I wanted them so I could put myself to sleep the way Dr. Martin did when Blackie got to be fifteen years old and was so crippled he couldn't even get up to pee. Would you still give me the prescription?"

"I'm afraid I couldn't. It's my duty as a doctor not to do anything to shorten life. People are not dogs."

"No, we aren't. But suppose I made out one of those living wills. Don't they say something about the doctor not using any 'extraordinary or heroic measures' to prolong life? Could you put me out then?"

"That doesn't help me much. A living will is like the Constitution — looks great on paper, but it can mean anything you want it to. What is an extraordinary measure? Antibiotics? Intravenous fluids? Spoon feeding? As to heroic measures, I promise you that if a bear breaks into your room and threatens to carry you off, I won't interfere."

"Then I'll put in my living will that I don't want you to do anything except give me medicine for pain. How would that be?"

"That would be fine. In that case, I would just be carrying out your wishes. A patient always has the right to refuse treatment."

"Even if I put down that I don't want you to try to resuscitate me if I came in with an overdose of sleeping pills?"

"That's a complicated issue. I'm not sure the living will covers suicide attempts."

"Life is complicated, Dr. Conger. But it's my life, after all. At least, I'm the major stockholder, I hope. And I want to finish it up right. I'll be darned if I'm going to hang around until people regret that I'm still alive. I want them to remember good old Merry, not some Skin-and-Bones Dunham. I won't ask you to kill me; just knock me out. A smart doctor like you shouldn't have trouble telling the difference between asleep and dead. Unless —Hypothermia! I know Mr. Shiftley has been trying to save on heating bills. Is it that cold up there?" From anyone else, I would have thought this last question was sarcastic, but Merry was just wondering.

"Can't you at least promise to give me enough medicine to put me to sleep human-style?"

"I guess I could do that."

"Well, then, that takes care of it. Don't worry," she added, noticing my startled expression. "Everything will turn out fine."

"Don't you want to know about treatment?" I was completely taken aback by her lack of interest in what I could do for her.

"I don't think so. A person of 'my age,' as you so diplomatically put it, shouldn't waste either of our time with procrastination. But it's sweet of you to offer."

"I just didn't want you to lose hope."

"I'm not worried about losing hope. What I don't want to lose is control."

"You didn't ask me how you happened to get cancer," I said, changing the subject. "Many people wonder about that."

"Just my luck, I suppose. Something has to get you."

"Not exactly. Statistics show that lung cancer occurs much more commonly in smokers."

I regretted the comment almost before it escaped my lips. The fact that Merry had been a smoker was of no relevance now, but I had to try something to establish control over a meeting that had up to this point been on Merry's terms. I should have known better.

"Statistics show lots of things. One out of every ten smokers will develop cancer in the course of their lifetime. When you stop to think about it, the amazing thing is not that so many people get cancer, but that we all don't get it. The lung makes about one hundred million cells every day. Each one of those cells is equipped with twenty thousand pairs of genes. One of those genes is called an oncogene. Oncogenes are used by the embryo to help it develop. At birth the oncogenes are locked up in a closet. Sometimes, however, the door pops open accidentally, and the oncogene gets turned on again. When this happens, the cells go haywire. It's hard to make things perfect. I can hardly complain if the system slips up once in every two trillion tries."

"I suppose not."

"No. You've been such a help, Dr. Conger. I'll be in

touch. Well, then, I'm off. Ta-ta." Merry patted me on the hand and, with a cheery wave, exited the premises.

Merry was fine for six months. She reorganized her committees. She made quilts for her nieces and nephews. She sorted out her books, donating to the library the ones it could use and giving away the rest to children. Then she took a holiday in the Caribbean. She had put this project off until last. "It's better to die with a tan," she said. "Less depressing to look at." She got back in the middle of April. She never left the house again. She didn't have to: everybody flocked to Merry's. Casseroles piled up in the freezer. Her floors were washed twice a day. Flowers appeared in such profusion that Merry said it looked as if she were having a funeral first and the death after. Billy Snide even brought her breakfast. All the attention wore on her, but she didn't say anything. She didn't want to upset anybody. Then five o'clock one morning she called.

"I'm sorry to bother you at this hour, Dr. Conger, but I think the time has come."

I met her at the hospital. She was drawn and tired. But her tan looked fine.

"It's been tough, hasn't it?" I commiserated.

"Oh, no!" she whispered. "It couldn't have been better. I had time enough to do everything I wanted. And I've got my pass to get me straight to the pearly gates without waiting in line. If you ask me, it's the only way to go." She stopped to catch her breath. "My, how hard it is to talk. That surely means the end, don't you think?"

"In your case, Merry, I would have to say yes."

"No point shilly-shallying around. You haven't forgotten your promise?"

I hadn't. I said good-bye. I gave her an injection of morphine. She fell asleep. Then I started an intravenous with enough morphine in the bottle to ensure that she wouldn't wake up. She slept peacefully for two days. On the third morning she died.

Merry was a good person. And a very good teacher. I only wish I had been a more attentive pupil.

17

There is an expression commonly seen on the faces of young people when they are listening to an edifying dissertation by some older and wiser person. The furrowed brow, bulging eyes, and tightened lips impart to the one who is speaking an impression that the listener is in a state of extreme concentration. To a more dispassionate onlooker, it might convey a sense of someone in great pain. Both observations are correct, for the younger in this instance is straining prodigiously to maintain the appearance of interest in the words of the elder, hoping that by so doing, the enlightenment at hand will be brought to a speedy conclusion.

It was precisely this expression that I beheld on the face of Sandra Smart, Dartmouth Medical School III, while I lectured to her about Fusswood's current malaise.

Once a year I have occasion to receive a medical student from Dartmouth in my practice. The curriculum guide states that the purpose of this sojourn is to

> give the student an opportunity to observe a non-academic, community-based practice and gain in-

sight into the issues involved in providing quality
medical care in such a setting.

In short, it is a chance to observe the natives in their
natural habitat. For me, the opportunity to participate,
however modestly, in shaping the doctors of tomorrow is an
honor bestowed upon me eagerly by a beleaguered medical
school, which is grateful that I am willing to provide them
with a temporary respite from these insatiable fledglings. As
reward, I am granted the rank of Supernumerary Instructor of Community Medicine, a title that brings with it a free
library card and reduced-rate parking at Mary Hitchcock
Hospital. For the students, the chance to work side by side
with a doctor who practices in the real world is considered
cruel and unusual punishment.

I can hardly blame them. I felt the same way when I was
as smart as they. But now, having risen eighteen years ago
from the seat of learning, my pearls of wisdom are so tar-
nished as to be of little value in today's marketplace of ideas.

Both Sandra and I knew that she had far more to teach
me than I her. Nevertheless, custom dictated that we act as
if the opposite were true. The object over which we were
currently carrying out this charade was Fusswood's right big
toe. Fusswood had experienced some difficulties with the
appendage recently and had brought it in for repair.

"I was sitting in the chair last night," he said, "and it gave
out a loud twang. Could hardly walk on it for twenty minutes. If you don't do something fast, I could wind up a
cripple. I don't mind telling you, Doc, I'm worrying."

"And so you should," I had replied after examining the
digit in question — a digit, I might add, that did not appear
to share in the least Fusswood's alarm over the recent turn
of events. "I suggest ten minutes of fretting about your tax
return after each meal and one serious panic about impo-
tence at bedtime. That should take care of things."

"Suppose it doesn't?"

"Then I'll chop it off. Now run along and get a urine sample. Let's see how the old kidneys are behaving today."

Fusswood trotted obediently off to the bathroom. Sandra turned to me aghast. "What if he should think you were serious?"

"Fortunately, I no longer have that problem."

———◄•►———

SERIOUS READER NOTE: Of all the diseases a physician may contract in the line of duty, by far the most dangerous is seriosity. Seriosity is a pervasive disease. It may appear as early as the first year of medical school in the industrious student who shuns the chance for a spring tan or an afternoon nap in favor of an intimate tête-à-tête with Gray's Anatomy. *During internship and residency, seriosity reaches epidemic proportions. In the practicing physician it can pop up anywhere: in the surgeon who is compelled to snip at organs that have long since ceased to be a source of interest to their owners; in the cancer specialist who labors tirelessly to ensure that her patients survive long enough to receive their full complement of poisons. Even the lowly general practitioner is not immune. I know of a case where an otherwise sensible associate suddenly became obsessed with the need to inflict on his congregation a host of healthy habits that were far more effective in promoting misery than in their intended purpose of prolonging life.*

What causes seriosity? Excessive adulation stimulates hypertrophy in the sense of importance, which leads to a corresponding atrophy in the sense of humor. This in turn induces a delusional state in which the victim believes nothing worthwhile can be accomplished without his personal intervention.

Seriosity is easy to miss. Its symptoms are often mistakenly attributed to other causes. Dedication. Obsessive-compulsive personality. An unhappy home life. By the time it is recognized, the disease is usually so far advanced that it is highly resistant to treatment. Sensitive egos are unable to cope with the discovery that most of their efforts are irrelevant and many may be downright harmful. It is quite depressing. Nowhere does the ounce of prevention carry greater weight than in the treatment of this dread disease.

If you are a patient and suspect that your doctor is showing signs of seriosity, you can help her lick it. Here's how:

1. *No matter what she prescribes, tell her Anacin works better.*
2. *Bring a crossword puzzle to the office. Work on it during the visit.*
3. *When she tells you you weigh too much, tell her you know a hairdresser who could do wonders for her appearance.*
4. *In the middle of the examination, tell her you have to leave for your dog's voice lessons.*
5. *Tell her your chiropractor has nicer hands.*

What little doubt Sandra had of my professional abilities had vanished. "Is that why you told him he ought to worry?" she asked. "So he wouldn't believe you?"

"On the contrary. I am a firm believer in the value of worrying." At this point I launched into the dissertation that had caused Sandra such discomfort.

"But," she protested when I had finished, "Dr. Pontifact told us that worry is unhealthy. He said it interferes with phytohemagglutination of B lymphocytes."

"That's a good point, Sandra. However, one must consider as well the salutary effect it has on the A lymphocyte."

"A lymphocytes? The only lymphocytes I know of, Dr. Conger, are B and T. You know, bursal and thymic."

"Uh. Yes. Well. I wouldn't be concerned with that. There are other factors to consider in worry which are much more important than lymphocytes."

"Oh, I know. Worry stimulates endogenous catecholamines, interferes with the diurnal rhythm of hydroxycortisone, and depresses high-density lipoproteins. This raises blood pressure, increases stomach acid, and elevates cholesterol levels. Of course you know what that means." She finished with a slight inflection in her voice so that it was unclear whether her last statement was declarative or interrogatory. I opted for the former and indicated my agreement with a dignified nod.

———————————

SERIOUS READER NOTE: I was not taught about worry in medical school. It was one of those things that doctors are just supposed to know — like how to remove a splinter, or how long someone has to live.

Somewhere early in my internship, I saw a patient with a pain behind his right ear. I couldn't find anything wrong. "Don't worry about it," I told him. Two months later he came into the emergency room with an overdose of sleeping pills. After we brought him around, I asked him why he had tried to do himself in.

"I couldn't stand it anymore."

"Couldn't stand what?"

"Waiting for it to get me."

"Waiting for what to get you?"

"Whatever it was that was too far advanced for me to worry about."

That was the last time I told someone not to worry. For many years thereafter, when confronted with the issue, I simply changed the subject. When I moved to California, I found out that worry, being a natural emotion, was good for you. (As with all California truths, this one has a caveat. A person who gets in a stew about an event whose probability of occurrence is high is engaged in worry that serves no useful purpose. On the other hand, should the object of his bother be sufficiently unlikely as to be fanciful, its contemplation can be quite beneficial. There is no experience more soothing than the abolition of an anticipated fright.)

Now, I recommend worry for all my patients. For example, if Fusswood should come into my office with a lump, I know the most likely thing to be on his mind would be cancer. In this case, I might suggest that he worry instead about being struck by a fallen tree on the way to work. The task of devising alternate transportation strategies would keep him sufficiently occupied so as to distract him from his more immediate concern, and the end of each day would find him quite contented that he was still alive and well.

I looked at Sandra, and I started to get that feeling I always got when in the presence of one of these eager young medical minds — the doctors of tomorrow, who will be treating Fusswoods of the future, and to whom I will become the Old Doc Conger that Old Doc Franklin is to me. The feeling is not one of which I am proud, but I promised to lay all the cards on the table, and so I will.

I hate medical students. They make me feel dumb, disorganized, and decrepit. With but a single slash of their tongues, these whippersnappers, still wet behind the stethoscope, can rend the canvas of my medical art and destroy the masterpiece I have spent years painstakingly creating, stroke by trial-and-error stroke. What do they know about the difficulties of practicing in a world where patients never get their symptoms right, and drugs don't remember which of their effects are side dishes and which the main course? Sandra knew her B lymphocytes and catecholamines. But did she know life? Maybe it was time to give her a lesson. One that would teach her a little respect for the life of an L.M.D.

———————◄•►———————

SERIOUS READER NOTE: L.M.D. Local Medical Doctor. The term is used in academic medicine to identify those physicians who practice outside the ivory tower. In the hierarchy of medical specialists, L.M.D.'s rank just above witch doctors. In the medical center they are seen as degenerates whose management of patients is so incompetent as to constitute quackery. Whenever a patient arrives at a teaching center on referral from an L.M.D., the first thing that is done is to congratulate him for having made the trip safely. Then the scurrilous information that has accompanied him is promptly discarded, and his evaluation begins from scratch.

Where do these incompetents get their education? From mail-order medical schools? From witch doctors, chiropractors, and the tales of old spouses? From Caribbean cabañas? No, on all counts. Strange as it may seem, these bumbling idiots have learned their trade in those very same citadels of learning that now so cruelly scorn them. They are none other than those whom their detractors will someday become.

———————◄•►———————

"You seem to have an excellent grasp of the issues involved in this case, Sandra. When Fusswood comes back, I'm going to let you take over."

"Me? Can I? Golly! This would be the first . . . I mean, I've never talked to a real patient before. I hope I can do it."

"Don't worry," I said, congratulating myself on the wisdom of my decision. "It's easy. Just pretend you're talking to a person."

"There is one thing I . . . Do you think . . . ? I mean, would it be OK . . . ? Well, we just had a lecture on Stress Management Theory, and — "

"You'd like to try it out on Fusswood?"

"Oh, yes! That is, if you don't think it would be contra-indicated."

"Not at all." I hadn't the foggiest notion what stress management was, but it sounded like the kind of impractical academic drivel that would be sure to land her right where I wanted her: in the soup. "Just what I was considering myself."

When Fusswood returned, Sandra greeted him.

"Good morning, Mr. Fusswood. My name is Sandra Smart. Dr. Conger has allowed me to work with you on your problem. I would like to employ a treatment called stress management. I think it can help solve your problem, but it will involve asking you some personal questions. Are you willing to try it?"

"Er, I guess so." Fusswood, unaccustomed to having his opinion asked, looked at me uncertainly. I nodded approval. "Sure. Why not?"

"We will start with a review of your current stress investments. This is a crucial component to any effective stress-management system. Your most important investment is, of course, your wife. Tell me, if you will, how much time you spend together."

"We go for long walks on Sunday afternoon, and we take each other out to dinner every other Friday."

"That's very good. How well would you say the two of you are getting along?"

"All in all, not too badly. But Martha complains that I never talk to her, and I get in a tizz trying to figure out what to say whenever she says, 'Talk to me!' "

"Hmmm. Communications down. How are things at work?"

"Until recently, lousy. I've been staying late at the office and bringing work home with me at night. Now, I'm less of a workaholic. Only problem is, the boss is threatening to block my promotion because he thinks I'm slacking off."

"Industrials fluctuating. What about your leisure-time activities?"

"I used to play so much golf, Martha said she was a golfing widow. So I cut back to once a week. After all, it's only a game."

"That's a very healthy attitude."

"Yeah, but what with less time at work and less time at golf, I spend a lot more time around the house."

"That should help you and Martha increase the return on your togetherness bonds."

"It doesn't. Martha says I'm poaching on her self-actualization time and stifling her individual expression. And she wants to watch *Days of Our Lives,* while I like *All My Children.*"

"I see. That is a problem. Well, there's no doubt your stress portfolio needs major adjustments. First, I would suggest purchasing additional shares in mutual interests. The easiest way to do this would be to buy a VCR. Then you can tape one soap while you watch the other. Afterward, you can discuss them over tea. That should improve considerably the value of both your togetherness and communications holdings.

"To balance this, Martha will need an outside interest. The simplest thing would be for you to divest your golf shares and transfer them to her.

"Finally, you need to convert your work stocks into boss anger futures. This is an excellent investment for those with excess stress capital."

"And if I do all this, my worries will be over?"

"Worries, yes. Stress, no. Stress is not like worry. You can never get rid of it. You manage it, so that it works for you instead of against you. It may take some time, but with proper attention, your medical concerns should become much less anxiety-provoking. To maximize the benefits, however, you should update your portfolio on a regular basis — if that meets with Dr. Conger's approval, of course."

It did.

"I guess that's it, then. It's been a real pleasure, Mr. Fusswood. I hope I've been of some help."

"More than you can imagine. You know, Doc, you've got a pretty sharp partner here. Might even teach you a few tricks. Well, Doc," he said, turning this time to Sandra, "nice meeting you. And good luck — not that you'll need it." With a smile at Sandra and a wink at me, Fusswood left.

Sandra could hardly contain herself. "Did you hear what he called me? Doc! Wow! I owe you an apology, Dr. Conger. All this time I thought general practice was so boring and you L.M.D.'s — I mean family doctors — were practicing medicine in the Stone Age. But I was wrong. This is what medicine is all about. Helping people. And you have so much to teach. Golly, maybe someday I can practice right here in Dumster. Just like you." Suddenly, her bubble burst. She turned to me hesitantly. "You will let me try another case, won't you?"

"Of course. That's what you're here for. I do have one suggestion before we see our next patient. It concerns how you introduce yourself."

"You mean I can say Dr. Smart? That would be fantas — No. That's not right. I'm not a real doctor yet, so I shouldn't call myself one."

"Quite right. I was going to suggest that it might be more appropriate for you to use an alias."

⚡ *18* ⚡

"*Strike one.*"
The crowd moved to the edge of their seats. A buzz swept through the stands.

"Strike two."

The buzz became a roar. It was the last inning. Two outs, bases loaded, three and two on the batter, and the Red Sox leading the Yankees two to one. What could be the last Yankee stepped back from the plate to tap some nonexistent dirt from the cleats. Having gained therefrom the requisite modicum of courage, the batter returned to the battlefield. The pitcher looked in. He shook his head once. Twice. He nodded. Then came the windup. And the pitch. The batter let it go. All eyes turned to the man in blue. For a second the arbiter was motionless. Then, he motioned for the ball. Up into the air went his right hand. Up onto its feet went the crowd. Up upon the tee went the ball. The batter swung. Skyward sailed the ball. His back pressed against the wall, the centerfielder raised his glove to the heavens as if in supplication. Like a bird of prey spotting its victim, the ball plummeted toward the glove. It struck the webbing, wobbled briefly, and disappeared into the pocket. An ecstatic crowd erupted onto the field. The fielder was transfixed, rooted to the spot by the weight of his victory spoils.

Equally immobilized at home plate was the batter. Both were dumbfounded by the mysterious forces that propelled this small white sphere from the one to the other, but both were equally convinced that the event was not the result of any act of volition on either of their parts. Gradually the full meaning of what had just transpired dawned upon the two combatants. One jumped into the air and let out a mighty whoop. The other sat down and cried.

I watched the vanquished batter rise slowly from the ground. Briefly our eyes made contact and then turned away — mine in guilt, hers in anger. Had it not been for her father, who insisted that if she wanted to play Little League it would be for the Yankees or not at all, the cheers could have been for her.

The sun shone brightly. The temperature was in the mid-eighties. It was one of those late May days that is a harbinger of the summer swelters. Perhaps it was the heat. Maybe the excitement. While I sat in the now empty stands, I became aware of a slight pressure in the back of my head. I looked in vain across the Dumster Fairgrounds for a spot of shade where I might take refuge from the sun. The pressure increased, tightening around my head like a steel band. I felt dizzy. A cold chill of fear made me shiver. Was this it? The end of a life I was just beginning to get the hang of? I had always said that I wanted to die before I got to that stage where a person can no longer remember that he doesn't want to be here, but forty-four seemed to be erring a little on the conservative side. At least it would be quick. I sat very still, waiting for proof that the little bubble inside my brain had burst. Nausea. Double vision. Confusion. Coma. Instead, my hand rose involuntarily to a point about six inches in front of what used to be my hairline. It paused for an instant and then jerked downward.

*   *   *

I tugged at my cap to block out the afternoon sun. It was a Yankee cap, it was two years old, and it was too tight, but since I had missed Cap Day that year, its retirement had been postponed until the next season. It was hot, and I was tired. I had been playing ball since eight that morning, stopping only briefly to run home for my three-pb-and-j lunch. Behind me were the Cliffs, a small outcrop of rocks that bordered the back of Soldiers and Sailors Field. Any ball hit into the Cliffs was an automatic homer. As the pitcher started his delivery, I pounded my glove in nervous anticipation.

I had never played against Billy Ryan. His home field was across town at the Rozelle Avenue Playground. Billy was the youngest of the three Ryan boys. His oldest brother, Joe, had just signed with the Yankees. Jerry was all-league short-shop for Pleasantville High School. Word was that Billy would be the best of the lot.

I could tell by the sound that it was a well-hit ball. Turning my back to the plate, I headed at full gallop toward the Cliffs. Just before crashing into what would have been the fence except that the fence wouldn't be erected for another two years, I saw a white blur in the sky. I reached out to grab it. The blur turned black.

"Is he dead?"

"Naw, I saw him twitch. It's just a combustion. See, he's opening his eyes."

"Hey, Chip. You OK? Ohmigod! What a catch! A Willie Mays!"

As the fog lifted from about my brain, I opened my eyes and looked down. Sure enough, there it was. Tucked safely in the pocket of my glove. The ball. Slowly I got up and limped off the field, shrugging off the offers of help. After all, I had just made my first over-the-shoulder catch.

I was first up next inning. Billy, who was playing third base, walked out to the mound and motioned for the ball. His first pitch was very fast. I let it go by, using the opportunity to set my swing for the next one. I needn't have bothered. The second pitch came straight at my head. In one of those split seconds that lasts forever, I remembered of Tony Cannizzaro. Tony was batting in the league championship for Pleasantville High School two years ago when an errant brush back hit him between the eyes. Since Tony's father didn't have insurance, the town raised the money for his three operations — and did so in a way that no Pleasantville kid will ever forget: it held a baseball game between the Pleasantville High Panthers and the New York Yankees, a game in which Mickey Mantle hit the ball not only out of the park, but across the brook and over the Saw Mill River Parkway. And Pleasantville's Ted Mazurowsky struck out Vic Raschi, who may only have been a pitcher but was still a Yankee. Despite the operations, Tony still can't see out of his right eye, and his left leg drags when he walks.

I was spared Tony's fate — not because I ducked, but because, when it was twenty feet from me, the ball took a sharp left turn and drifted harmlessly across the middle of the plate.

I got up and dusted myself off. I tossed my bat away. Then I tucked my cap in my back pocket and walked off the field. My baseball career was over. One look at that pitch was enough to tell me that between the some who can and the rest who can't, the former was not to be my gang. I would never be able to hit a curve.

In 1954, a thirteen-year-old boy who was too small for football and couldn't dribble with both hands didn't have many options left in the athletic division of pubertal rites.

So I became a runner.

In 1954 runners didn't have their own shoes or their own pants. In 1954 running was considered boring, painful, and useless. In 1954 the only people who ran were those who were in trouble. In 1954 the Boston Marathon had two hundred entrants.

Today people are running all over the place. They run to work. They run at night. They run in the snow. They run on television. Runners have their own clubs and their own stores. There are even books about running.

I still run. Not because I like it all that much, but because I'm afraid to stop. As a consequence, I have become a "runner's doctor." Other runners, knowing that I am likely to be more understanding, come to me with their problems. This was why I got a call from Sam Binder when he heard that Jim Fixx had died.

Ordinarily the news that a man had died in the woods of Vermont would excite no more interest than if one had dropped dead on the streets of New York, both being locations where the respective inhabitants thereof spend a considerable portion of their waking hours.

However, when James Fixx died from a heart attack in Hardwick, Vermont, it made the front page of the *New York Times*. Mr. Fixx was the author of a popular book on running. It is one of many current works that provide instruction on the proper performance of normal bodily functions. The book contains everything a runner needs to know. It has practical advice, such as how to tie your shoelaces to minimize wind resistance. It has information on what food runners should eat, what air runners should breathe, and what music runners should listen to. It even has a section on God's favorite running trails.

It was not, however, his authorship alone that put Mr. Fixx on page one. It was the fact that he died while running. This is not supposed to happen. Running is good for people. The reason we know this to be true is that it is so unpleasant.

If a runner is to die running, it should be because he has been run over by a truck. He should not have a heart attack. The death of Jim Fixx posed a serious threat to all runners, who depend on running for preservation of their illusion of immortality.

Sam Binder is fifty-five years old. In his former life he ate too much, smoked too much, and exercised not at all. Now he is a born-again runner. When he called me he was terrified.

"Hey, Doc, did you hear about Jim Fixx?"

"Sure did, Sam. Just one of those things. We've all got to go sometime. Could just as easily have happened while he was buttering his toast. I don't think it's anything to be alarmed about."

"But he was running! It said in the paper that he had a family history of heart trouble. My grandmother died of a coronary. And she was a woman, Doc! I'm in serious trouble."

"How old was she?"

"Eighty-nine. But that's not the point. Once you got it in the family, you never know where it's going to hit. You told me running would take care of me. What am I going to do now?"

"Stop running."

"Don't say that. When I broke my ankle, and I had to quit for two weeks, I got headaches, put on thirty pounds, and was so depressed I didn't care."

"Hmm. Running Withdrawal Syndrome. Sounds like you're hooked. Well, if you can't run less, there's only one other choice."

"What's that?"

"Run more."

"I'm already running thirty miles a week."

"George Sheehan went over Jim Fixx's mileage logs himself. It turns out the guy was all talk and no action. He was only doing twenty miles per, and he hadn't finished a marathon in over a year. No wonder he croaked."

"Forty, huh? I guess thirty miles isn't much better."

"A drop in the bucket. For a guy in your situation, who wants full cardiac protection, I'd say you better take her right on up to eighty, with three marathons and at least one ultra every year. I've never seen a ticker on that kind of schedule cause any trouble."

"Consider it done, Doc. But when Betty complains about not seeing me, I'm sending her to you."

"Just tell her you're trying to protect her investment."

"Good idea. Thanks a mill. I knew I could count on you to come up with something."

"That's my job, Sam. Now get out there and save that heart."

"I'm on my way."

———◄ ♦ ►———

Serious reader note: In 1924, the Western Electric Company hired a man by the name of C. E. Snow to figure out how much illumination it took to ensure maximum productivity on its assembly lines. C.E. studied the women who wound induction coils at the Hawthorne Electric Works in Cicero, Illinois. He started off by increasing the lighting from twenty-four to forty-eight footcandles. The women wound faster. Western Electric decided that the cost of extra electricity was well worth the increase in induction-coil output. They were very pleased with the findings. C E. Snow was not. He went back to the factory and changed the lights again — only this time he reduced the power to eighteen footcandles. To his surprise, the women wound faster again. He told Western Electric. They were ecstatic. C. E. Snow was not. He couldn't understand what was going on. So he tried one last experiment. He went into the room where the women were working and made a big fuss about changing the light bulbs. He told everyone how these bulbs were the latest thing in induction-coil-winding lights, and how, although he couldn't promise it, the lights would not only make them work faster and earn more money, but also just might help them lose weight and prevent the common cold. The lights he put in were exactly the same as the ones he took out. When he turned them on, the women wound their coils faster than ever before.

C. E. Snow got a lot of credit for his observation, which is now called the Hawthorne effect. But he was not the one who discovered it. Doctors have recognized the phenomenon for thousands of years as the "fuss factor." It is the cornerstone of medical practice. In days of yore, the fuss factor was administered with leeches and laxatives. Today the techniques are much more sophisticated, but the principle remains the same. If a patient is feeling poorly, in order to get credit for making him better, the doctor must do something. The precise nature of the something does not really matter, as long as he does it.

It might be a laboratory test. The patient who complains of a stomach ache, for example, could get a colonoscopy. Very few patients ever complain about their stomach after having a colonoscopy.

It might be a pill.

It might be an operation. Twenty years ago there was an operation for coronary disease called internal mammary artery implantation. The operation involved taking an artery that ran on the underside of the breast bone, cutting it off at one end, and sticking it into the heart. It was very popular in its day. But some surgeons were skeptical about whether this procedure actually improved blood flow to the heart. So they selected a group of patients who were planning to have the operation and divided them into two groups. On the first group they did the standard internal mammary artery implantation. They brought the second group to the operating room and made a long incision in the skin, just as they would for an implantation. At this point, however, they changed the procedure slightly. Instead of opening up the chest and implanting the artery *in the heart, they closed the skin and sent the patient back to the recovery room. Both groups of patients got excellent relief from their angina. The surgeons concluded that the internal mammary artery implantation was no good because the so-called sham operation did just as well.*

It was a good study, but they reached the wrong conclusion. What it really showed is that there's no such thing as an operation that doesn't work.

19

"*I can't believe it!*"

"What?"

"That he would pull a stunt like this!"

"Who?"

"Him!" Sarah shoved the sheet of paper in my face.

MEMORANDUM

TO: All nursing personnel
FROM: Herbert Shiftley, Administrator
DATE: June 5, 1986
RE: Working hours

Effective July 1, nursing shifts will be as follows:
    First shift: 7 AM–7 PM
    Second shift: 7 PM–7 AM

To ensure equitable assignment of working hours, nurses will alternate shifts every two weeks.

I regret any inconvenience this may cause.

"Gee, that's too bad. But I guess he doesn't have much choice."

"Outrageous is what it is. He's got plenty of choice."

This unexpected display of emotion by Sarah startled me. I had never seen her this animated. In the hospital forest, the Red-cheeked Angrynurse is a most uncommon bird, and he who spots one has made a rare sighting indeed. So infrequently is it seen that its appearance rivals in notability that of the Droop-shouldered Humbledoc. But there could be no mistake: Sarah was upset.

I could understand her feelings. It was difficult, especially for a single parent — as many of her colleagues were — to have her schedule so suddenly disrupted. But it struck me that Sarah's attitude was not completely proper. This was, after all, a hospital. And a hospital had to have nurses. The fact that there was currently a shortage of intelligent, compassionate souls who were willing to throw their lives away on the ungrateful sick was not Shiftley's fault. He was not a bad chap, after all, and I was sure he would never do such a thing if it wasn't absolutely necessary. I was about to explain this to Sarah, when something about her look made me hesitate.

"Why would he —"

"Pull a stunt like this without consulting us? I'll tell you why. Because he's chicken! Last week five nurses quit. Three of them went to work at Mary Hitchcock, where they got a dollar-an-hour raise, and the others are at home with their kids. They figured that five seventy-five an hour, once you finished paying for child care, therapy, and Tagamet, wasn't worth the hassle. Shiftley gave the rest of us a pep talk at one of his Employee Chats, as he calls them — Shiftley's Shifties is what they are — that we nurses were the 'vital organ of the hospital body.' So what does he do? Yesterday he had the nerve — no, he hasn't got any nerves. He had the . . ." — she sputtered at her inability to find the right epithet —"whatever, to tell us that the trustees had voted to 'defer' our raises for six months because the hospital was 'experiencing reimbursement delays' and 'cash-flow shortfalls.' Then he asked us to all 'pull together in this, our hour of greatest strife.' And when Ellen Blum asked him about the day-care center for employees — which he had agreed to provide space for — he changed the subject. I'll tell you one thing: if he doesn't get some treatment for his precious 'vital organ' pretty quick, it's going to —"

"Organize?" While Sarah was conducting her diatribe, the vague shadow of unease, which had appeared at the start of our conversation, was taking on a more distinct shape. The shape of guilt. As physician representative to the board of trustees, an honor traditionally accorded the most junior member of the medical staff, I had been present when the discussion she referred to had taken place. Herb had given an eloquent speech about the problems caused by delays in getting money from Medicare and the need to preserve the two-million-dollar endowment to help finance the hospital expansion, which was now trimmed down to bare essentials. He had eliminated the patient lounge and employee day-care center, so that all that was left was the administrative offices and doctors' cafeteria. Furthermore, he said, he had decided not to take his own raise until October, and he was going to ask the staff to join with him in this sacrifice. At the time, I thought it sounded fair enough. After all, he needed an office. The doctors had no place to go to escape the noisy atmosphere at the nurses' station. And he was asking no more of the nurses than he was of himself, although a pay freeze at forty thousand dollars a year is not quite the same as one at fourteen, especially with the possibility of a big bonus at the end of the year should the hospital turn out in the black.

SERIOUS READER NOTE: It is a peculiar paradox of the medical industry that hospitals, which, with a few exceptions, are not businesses, pretend devoutly that they are; while doctors, who are the profit motive incarnate, pretend just as earnestly that they are not. As a consequence, hospitals are always fussing about their "bottom line," which is so far down in the financial well full of endowments, fund raisings, and cost shiftings as to be unfathomable. And doctors steadfastly refuse to admit that any of their actions have a substantial effect not just on the health of their patients' bodies, but on the welfare of their respective pockets as well.

"Don't be silly. I'm not trying to cause trouble. I just want us to get what's fair."

"You'll never get what you deserve if you don't organize. Have you forgotten the lessons of the 'sixties?"

"In the 'sixties I was working days to raise the kids and working nights to put Jeff through medical school. I didn't have time for lessons. Let's see. I suppose what we should do is join the Teamsters, boycott the cafeteria, and hold a protest vigil in Mr. Shiftley's office."

There was a certain tone in her voice that kept me from saying that these were exactly the steps I had in mind. A tone that indicated Sarah was in need of a little consciousness raising.

"Why don't you come to the next meeting of Physicians for Social Responsibility? It might lend you some inspiration."

"Isn't that the antinuclear group? I don't see how they can help us."

"Never underestimate the power of physicians."

Sarah said she couldn't argue with that, and she agreed to come, although I wasn't sure if it was because she wanted to see what they had to say or figured it was the only way to shut me up.

I love to cause trouble. If there's something I can do to set a quiet pot boiling, I will be on it in a flash. And if the particular pot in question happens to be a worthy one, so much the better. It's not often that I get such an opportunity. I was born a multihandicapped child. White. Middle-class. Anglo-Saxon. Male. Participation in the plight of the oppressed has not come easy. As a child, the best I could do was sell Girl Scout cookies for my sister. College was not much better. I was far removed from the urban civil rights action, and I went to school before the Vietnam war had been discovered. I was forced to content myself with writing scathing letters to the student newspaper about social myopia among the academic elite.

It wasn't until medical school that I got a chance to try my hand at some serious do-gooding. In my second year I ran into a professor named Jack Leeder. He had been a journalist but switched to medicine when he discovered that doctors made better crusaders than newspaper readers. His cause was health for the poor, the banner around which he rallied read "Medical Committee for Human Rights," and the message he whispered was "Health is power. Power to the people." Dr. Leeder was a devout believer in people. Provided, of course, that the people had proper direction. That was where the Medical Committee for Human Rights came in. The year was 1964. Congress had just declared war on poverty, and the federal government was gearing up its mighty war machine to do battle. Dr. Leeder was the admiral of a brand-new fleet of poverty-blasting warships that were intended to take the fight to the enemy on its home front. Leading the assault was a magnificent battleship designed and built by Dr. Leeder himself. The U.S.S. *Neighborhood Health Center*. It was a mighty vessel indeed. Its deck bristled with the latest in poverty-fighting weaponry: disease-seeking statistics, multiwarhead prevention plans, interdisciplinary ballistic organizers. Dr. Leeder was eager to put his ship into battle, but, like any prudent commander, he wanted to ensure that it met with success on its first outing, so that its highly motivated, but as yet untested, crew would not become discouraged by some unexpected adversity and give up the fight before it had even begun. After scouting the Boston area for several months, he found the perfect target: the town of Lexington.

Lexington, Mississippi, is the capital of Holmes County, the only county in Mississippi with a large enough population of blacks who were sufficiently independent that they would be able to withstand the devastating crossfire that would inevitably erupt when the Holmes County whites found out what was going on. Except for the director, the administrator, and the professional staff, the ship would be run completely by a local crew.

I volunteered to be one of the advance troops. Our job was to soften up the opposition with an undercover hit-and-run guerrilla action that would elevate health awareness among the native poor and make them eager for insurrection when the liberation forces arrived. There was reason to believe that in Holmes County, health was not considered to be a high-priority item on the list of life's troubles. When asked how we were to go about accomplishing our assignment, Dr. Leeder was not specific, but he emphasized that we were of crucial importance to the success of the mission.

Upon arriving in Mississippi, I reported to the office of the Student Nonviolent Coordinating Committee. The Medical Committee for Human Rights, not yet having established diplomatic relations with Mississippi, conducted its activities through the SNCC embassy. After giving me a cursory and, I felt, not entirely complimentary appraisal, the field director handed me a large manila folder. "There's a map inside. It has directions to the place you'll be staying. The area shaded in gray is your territory. Pink forms are voter registration. Yellow ones are school applications. I assume you can tell who needs which. Turn them in here once a week. There are three rules: Walk facing traffic. Never ride with a black in front. Keep a dime inside your shoe. They allow you one call, but you have to pay for it." With my orientation completed, he returned to the conversation my arrival had interrupted.

"Excuse me, Mr. Lewis," I said. "I think there's been a slight mistake. You see, I am Dr. Conger." I used the title only to emphasize my intended role. "I was sent by the Medical Committee for Human Rights to organize health care."

"There's been a mistake, all right. It was made by the bozo who thought we needed Band-Aids when we can't vote or go to a decent school. This is the work. If you want to help, take it. Otherwise, get out."

I took it. It was a hard summer. I was harried. I was harassed. I was helpless. And I didn't do a damn bit of good to anyone. But it was worth it. By the time I got back to Boston, I had become a genuine agitator. So, when I became an intern at Boston City Hospital, and I joined — however temporarily — a bona fide oppressed minority, I was ready. The cause at hand was honest enough: decent wages and reasonable working conditions. When the city refused to accede to our demands — five hundred dollars a month in salary, technicians to do lab tests we ordered so we could spend as much time caring for patients as we did cleaning test tubes, and at least one nurse to cover every ward so we wouldn't have to dispense our own pills on Saturday night — we took action. A strike, we figured, wasn't exactly ethical. We had a heal-in instead. It was very simple. All we did was refuse to discharge any patients. Within forty-eight hours the hospital was in chaos, and the city caved in. We got all our demands — except the nurses. A lot of them quit during the heal-in, and the city couldn't find replacements.

After that, things were pretty quiet until I discovered Physicians for Social Responsibility, an organization dedicated to the proposition that war, if it happened to be of the nuclear variety, is bad for a person's health.

Spaulding Auditorium at Dartmouth was packed. The speaker was Dr. Harriet Goodworth, a psychiatrist from Boston and an authority on the health implications of nuclear war. She had written numerous scientific articles on the subject and was the author of a best-selling book, *A Physician's Guide to Armageddon.*

"I don't need to remind you," she started, "that the United States and Soviet Union are engaged in a massive proliferation of nuclear arms that has already produced enough weapons to kill every human being on this planet one hundred times over." (A low rumble from the crowd.) "Despite this appalling fact, our government has steadfastly refused to acknowledge the medical catastrophe that would ensue should even a fraction of these weapons ever be used. President Reagan himself has declared that a nuclear war could be won, and the Department of Health, Education and Welfare has tried to minimize the risks of nuclear war by presenting it as just another natural disaster. I have here a booklet printed by our own surgeon general." (She held a small pamphlet over her head. Louder rumble.) "It is called *In Time of Emergency,* and it tells what we should do when the end is imminent. It contains such advice as 'Take cover instantly' and 'Never look at a fireball.' It's a must for every

home and office within fifty miles of a potential target."
(Laughter.)

"Our media are no better. They may be muckraking sen-
sationalists about the sexual proclivities of our politicians, but
when it comes to covering the Big Blast, they become mealy-
mouthed wimps." (Scattered boos.) "I'm sure all of you have
seen *The Day After*." (Chorus of assent.) "This purportedly
realistic film about the dropping of a hydrogen bomb on an
American city is such a gross understatement of the catastrophe that would ensue should nuclear war actually break
out as to make it suitable for inclusion in a book of fairy tales.
Assuming for a minute that the Soviet Union was considerate
enough to restrict its bombing to military targets, thereby
guaranteeing at least some survivors, what would it be like for
those of us who were still around to treat the victims?

"One single ICBM has a destructive force of one hundred
Hiroshima equivalents."

———◄ ► ———

*SERIOUS READER NOTE: One Hiroshima equivalent is three
hundred thousand people, the number killed when we bombed Hiroshima. Putting nuclear war in Hiroshima equivalents makes it
more comprehensible to the average person, who has trouble with
large numbers.*

———◄ ► ———

"Thirty million people would die outright." (Gasps.) "Do
you know how long it would take the surviving physicians
just to write thirty million death certificates?" (Silence.)
"Two weeks." (More gasps.)

"Another thirty million would be critically injured. We

would need, in order to provide proper treatment, one hundred and fifty million gallons of intravenous fluid, four billion milligrams of morphine, and fourteen million hours of nursing overtime. Where are we going to get it? From the White House?" (Loud boos.)

"Not that it really matters, because it would take all our ambulances two years to transport these patients to medical facilities. Which we couldn't do anyway, because there wouldn't be any gasoline. What does President Reagan expect us to do? Make house calls?" (Roars of laughter.)

"But the impact on humans is only a fraction of the total disaster picture. Heat from the blast would melt the ice cap and relocate the Atlantic Coast to somewhere west of Buffalo. Its firestorm would reduce the ozone layer so much that all animals not wearing sunglasses would be blinded. And the radiation would cause enough mutations to turn most animal and plant species into genetic monsters." (Cries of protest.)

"We have no time to lose! The Doomsday Clock stands at one minute to midnight and counting. A misguided finger could push the nuclear button at any moment. We must act now!" (Cheers.) "What, you ask, can we as doctors do? We can do plenty. Inside every government official who makes laws, inside every contractor who builds weapons, inside every soldier who uses them, even inside President Reagan, is a patient. Do you know what that means?" (Scattered yeses.) "Do you?" (A thunderous yes.) "Of course you do! Imagine this. Doctor is performing a colonoscopy on patient. The scope has slid around the splenic flexure and is heading for the transverse colon. Suddenly, doctor stops the procedure and addresses patient. 'Excuse me, Mr. President, while I've got your attention, there's something I'd like to ask you to do for the world.' " (Loud cheers and stomping of feet.) "If every doctor in this country — and I have assurances from our compatriots in the Soviet Union that, if we will only show the way, they are prepared to do the same — took just five minutes to speak to each of his patients about nuclear holocaust, we could not only turn back the hands on the Doomsday Clock, we could shut it off." (More cheers and stomping of feet.) "So what are you waiting for, doctors? Go out there and treat!" (Standing ovation with clapping, cheers, and whistles.)

Two days later, when I saw Sarah, I asked her what she thought of the lecture.

"If the International Brotherhood of Plumbers formed an organization called Plumbers for Social Responsibility, the primary goal of which was to educate the public about the plumbing implications of nuclear war — which, I suspect, are substantial — people would say they were pompous, arrogant, and a bunch of fools. Plumbers, fortunately, have more sense than that. Still, I'll admit Dr. Goodworth had a point."

"So what are you going to do about the situation?"

"Nothing."

"Nothing? You mean after all that?" I could hardly believe she had given up so easily. But a nurse is a nurse.

"There's no need to. Mr. Shiftley has agreed to give us a ten-percent raise, to make the shift changes optional, and he promised to convert the doctors' cafeteria into a day-care center. He's even talking about building an employee swimming pool. You know, this could be a pretty nice place to work."

"But —"

"He decided to do it himself. Right after I talked to him about how our patients always say it is we nurses who make the difference about what it's like to be in the hospital."

"That was all?"

"Yup. It was a very nice chat. Especially the part where I told him how much the nurses were looking forward to taking care of him when he came in for his hernia operation next week."

﹄ *20* ﹌

"**W**haa-at's up, Doc?"
He was dressed immaculately. Three-piece gray
worsted Brooks Brothers suit, pale yellow oxford shirt, and
sky-blue Gucci loafers. In his jacket pocket was a pink pais-
ley Christian Dior handkerchief that matched his tie, which
was held in place by a large gold stickpin. When we shook
hands, I got a discreet whiff of wild musk. Ralph looked like
someone you could trust. Someone who was on friendly
terms with money. He needed no introduction, but as it was
part of our greeting ritual, he handed me his card.

Ralph Eversby Pushpil
Professional and Educational Representative
MedTex Pharmaceuticals

Ralph Pushpil didn't consider himself a salesman. As
Ralph explained it, his job was not to peddle drugs, but to
serve as a resource to the doctor who was too busy to keep
up with the latest advances in pharmacotherapeutics, at
least that branch of pharmacotherapeutics that was repre-
sented by the MedTex Pharmaceutical Company.

I looked forward to my visits with Ralph. Pills, after all, were not only his business, they were mine too. He always popped up at the right time, just when the medicines I was using had either become so ineffective as to be useless, or too toxic even to try. His sense of timing was uncanny. It was almost as if he knew exactly when a particular drug would become obsolete. I was certainly ready for him when he showed up.

"What have you got for me today, Ralph?" I asked, trying to sneak a peek inside his display case, which he had just placed, slightly ajar, on my desk. "Something good, I hope."

"I got stuff here that will blow your mind. But first, take a look at this." He pulled out a long envelope and pushed it across the table to me. "Go ahead, open it."

Office of the President
MedTex Industries
"The People Pleasing Company"

Dear Doctor CONGER,

Congratulations! Because of your judicious use of the MedTex fine line of pharmaceutical products, you have been selected as DUMSTER's Doctor of the Year. In recognition of this honor, I am pleased to award you and your WIFE, TRINE, a one week all expense paid trip on the island of Grenada, where you will be staying as our guests at the lovely new Grenadier Hotel, another in the fine line of products from MedTex.

On behalf of MedTex, and your Professional and Educational Representative, RALPH PUSH-PIL, I hope you and your WIFE have a good time, and I want to thank you again for thinking of

MedTex in your patients' hours of medicinal need.

Your friend,
M. C. Fayerbrush
President

It was signed by Mr. Fayerbrush himself.

"Just a little token of our appreciation, Doc. Of course, if there's someone you'd rather take than the little lady" — he paused to accommodate a slight twitch in his left eye — "I can have the tickets changed in a jiff. It's all done by computer, you know."

"That won't be necessary. Trine would love to go," I said. "I must say, I'm touched. I never realized you folks cared so much." I didn't have the heart to tell him what Trine would say when she saw the tickets. As chair of the Family Integrity Board, she was not likely to understand this offer as simply a gesture of professional goodwill.

"Let's just say you scratch my back, and I scratch yours." He twitched again. Apparently Ralph had a tic. "But enough of this small talk. Let's get down to business. I would guess those antibiotics of yours have probably gotten pretty stale by now. Am I right?"

"You can say that again. The Kilabugger was great stuff — until pseudomonas and serratia became so resistant, you would have thought it was Miracle Gro. Then, when all my patients started bleeding like stuck pigs because it wiped out their platelets . . . well, I hate to admit it, but I went back to penicillin."

"Penicillin?" Ralph croaked, his usually mellifluous voice suddenly turned hoarse. "Why didn't you give me a call? A good customer — uh, Doctor, like you? We wouldn't leave you in a jam. I could have brought you some advance samples. We always got a batch available for preliminary marketing — testing — just to handle situations like this. But" — he eyed me suspiciously — "you know that."

"Well . . ." I hesitated, reluctant to admit that I had some misgivings about trying his latest offering on my already pharmacologically abused patients, then went on, "I didn't want to bother you."

"Bother. Bother? Sorry, afraid I don't know that word, Doc. Anyway. No use crying over spilt milk. Let me show you what you missed." He pulled out a multicolored brochure from his bag. It showed a picture of a distinguished-looking young doctor. On his face was an expression suggesting that he was quite pleased with himself. On the bed beside him was a young, attractive female patient. She was looking up at the doctor with what could only be considered, except by sex fiends, as an expression of gratitude. She was lying supine in her bed with her hand extended toward the doctor and was dressed in a lavender hospital gown, which for some inexplicable reason she had put on backward, so that it opened in the front. The caption read, "I don't know how I can ever thank you enough, Doctor CONGER. You and Costatoxin have saved my life."

"This Costatoxin is great stuff. Has the full spectrum of Kilabugger, but none of those pesky bleeding problems. It's guaranteed to kill all staph on sight. As for pseudomonas — they won't even know what hit them. And, get this, Doc. Here's the best part: for every ten doses, you get five bonus points."

As part of their professional relations, MedTex, like all the drug companies, offered bonus points, which a doctor accumulated by using their products. When a doctor had earned enough, he could cash them in for textbooks, diagnostic instruments, vintage wines, and other necessary medical equipment. The drug companies offered these as a public service to doctors, who were too busy to get these things themselves. They emphasized that in no way was this practice to be considered an inducement to prescribe their drugs.

"Sounds pretty good. I'd love to try it out. Only one thing, though."

"You want to know how much it costs? Don't be afraid to ask, Doc. I know how it is these days."

"It's not that I care personally, you understand. It's just that every time I turn around these days, there's Shiftley hollering about costs. At two hundred bucks a day, Kilabugger had him in a complete snit. And when we had to start giving fresh platelet transfusions, well, it was getting so that I was afraid to pass him in the hall. It's that damn prospective-payment system. He can't let the meter run the way they used to. A patient gets admitted, and the hospital gets paid, depending on the diagnosis, a flat fee regardless of how much it actually costs to take care of him. Every time I order a test or prescribe a drug, it's an out-of-pocket expense. Shiftley watches us doctors like a hawk. He's got a review board to evaluate whether the tests I order are necessary. And he even has people checking up to see if my patients really need to be in the hospital. It's a nightmare."

"I understand. But not to worry. Costatoxin costs only thirty dollars a dose. That's half the price of Kilabugger."

"Seems like a pretty reasonable price. What's the dosage schedule?"

"One gram every two hours."

"Great. Put us down for five kilos. I'll clear it with the pharmacy."

"That's my boy. Now I'm going to show you something that will blow your mind. Take a look at these babies." He pulled out of his bag half a dozen small bright-blue bottles on which was embossed, in bold gold letters, the word *Auranofin*. "They're worth their weight in gold."

"Come on now, Ralph. You're getting carried away."

"Couldn't be more serious if my life depended on it. This stuff is made of real gold. It's the latest thing for the discriminating arthritis victim. Once you've started your patients on Auranofin, you can kiss the nonsteroidals good-bye forever."

"Oral gold. That's quite a breakthrough. I suppose it's much less toxic than the injections." Intramuscular gold injections have been used for many years to treat advanced cases of rheumatoid arthritis. Although they are quite effective, they are also extremely toxic. Their application is usually restricted to very advanced cases.

"We've still got a few bugs to work out, but nothing for you to bother your hardworking head about. Just be sure to keep a close eye on the liver and kidneys. With those babies on the fritz, life can be nasty business. Well" — he snapped his case shut to indicate that today's session of Educational Representations had come to an end — "it's Hi-Ho-Silver-and-away time. Nice talking to you, Doc. If you run low on silver bullets, give a buzz."

"Good to see you, too, Ralph. Seems like there's a new drug out every week. It's so hard to keep up with them. I don't know what I'd do without your help."

"Don't mention it, Doc. The pleasure is all mine."

⤸ 21 ⤷

"*I*t's all a matter of proper eating," declared my father-in-law as he prepared to attack the food mountain before him. "Your body is a precision machine. To run properly it must have the right fuel. That's where you Americans get in trouble." On the mountain's peak was a raw egg. Arne stabbed it once with his fork. The yolk slithered down the slopes of raw hamburg until it reached the bottom, where it disappeared into the thick slice of buttered bread that lay at the base. This was *aftens,* the Norwegian bedtime snack.

"What you Yanks need to do," explained Arne, pausing in his discourse to take a swig of akevitt, "is eat more fish."

------◄•►------

SERIOUS READER NOTE: Norwegians are a very shy people. It is difficult for them to express themselves in front of strangers. This is why many people think that Norwegians are taciturn. They are not. Norwegians love nothing better than a good gab. However, before they can enter into any conversation other than that which serves an immediate practical need, they must first overcome their shyness. This they accomplish with akevitt.

Akevitt (from the Latin aqua vitae, *meaning "water of life") is a potent shyness-fighting drug. It is made from potatoes (not surprisingly), and it contains 40 percent alcohol.*

The process of making akevitt is quite unusual. Once the beverage has been distilled from its potato mash, it is placed in large wooden caskets and loaded onto Norwegian freighters in the capital city of Oslo. From here it is shipped halfway around the world to the land Down Under. When the freighters get to Australia, they turn around and bring their cargo back home. This kind of thing, which may seem strange to us, makes perfect sense to Norwegians, whose philosophy is best expressed in the old Norsk saying "Life is as hard as you make it." The fresh sea air, gentle rocking on the waves, and change in climate are said to improve the flavor of the beverage. Every bottle of akevitt has a red line around it to prove that it has made a voyage across the equator. Whether the trip does much for akevitt I don't know, for I have never tasted any that stayed at home, but it is very beneficial to the Norwegian shipping industry.

"Air," interjected Uncle Knut, punctuating his rebuttal with a wave of his cigarette, "is what you're lacking. Good clean air. Can't run a body without it."

"Fish," said Arne. "Norwegians eat fish with every meal, even breakfast. That's why we're so healthy."

"We start them at an early age. Norwegian babies are put into fresh Norwegian air as soon as they can breathe."

"And potatoes. Without potatoes, the fish is useless. Norwegians eat two kilos of potatoes every day."

"Even in the winter — especially in winter. That's when the air is freshest and most beneficial to the lungs. Lungs are very important for good health. I've seen pictures of American lungs. Black. Just like coal. You know why?" Knut coughed. "Air pollution."

SERIOUS READER NOTE: Norwegian conversation is not con-ducted like ordinary conversation, where one person listens to what another has to say and then gives a response that, even if it dis-agrees, acknowledges the argument of his partner. Norwegian con-versational style comes from their ancestors, the Vikings, who had a language with only twenty-seven words and communicated with one another by throwing stones, conveying subtle nuances of thought by varying the size, velocity, and target of the stone. In Norwegian conversation the principle is to rebut your opponent's argument by refusing to acknowledge that it exists; and to improve the weight of your own, should it be deficient in facts or logic, by using the less substantial but more bulky substitutes of repetition and magnifica-tion. With respect to the matter of proof (a matter that arises only when one of the two conversing parties is not Norwegian), there is but one response: "In Norway, we do it like that." This is not a factual observation. It is a logical premise that carries the same meaning for Norwegians as the statement "It is the will of Allah" would for a Moslem.

It is not the fault of the Norwegians that their communication skills are rather limited. Norway is a heavily wooded and sparsely populated land. Consequently, a Norwegian's best friend is usually a tree. Anyone who has tried to reason with a tree will understand why Norwegians speak the way they do.

Norwegians were officially converted to Christianity cen-turies ago. They were unstinting in their proclamations of love for Jesus Christ. But in their hearts they are still pa-gans, and their true objects of worship are the twin deities of their ancestors: air and fish.

Air. I have walked through the streets of Oslo in the dead

of winter, and I have seen thousands upon thousands of little Nordic babies out in the frigid arctic air. Babies bundled up in strollers. Babies pulled on sleds. Babies sitting on front porches. Babies hanging from windows. Seeing these quiet, lifeless babies — innocent tears frozen on their colorless cheeks, fingers brittle as tiny icicles — I have often wondered if it might not be some effect of this fresh air program on their tender little brains that explains many of the peculiarities of the Norwegians.

Fish. Fish is nutritious and simple to prepare. It is not difficult to fix a tasty meal of fish. But the children of Odin are a resourceful lot. Here are two of their favorite recipes for nature's gift from the sea:

1. Lutefisk: Take a fresh fish. Hang it outside your window in the fresh Norwegian air for two months. Stick it in a pot of Drāno for two days. Remove and garnish with horseradish before serving.
2. Rakefisk: Take another fish. Stick it in a pot of brine. Bury the pot in the ground for four months. Salt to taste, and serve.

Norway is a country where the climate and geography can be quite inhospitable. It takes a very special people to populate such a land — people who would not be tempted to pack their rucksacks and hop a jet for Hawaii with the first September snow. Norwegians take great pains to ensure that each new generation inherits the cultural values that foster appreciation of Norwegian life. Trine, having moved to San Diego at age eighteen and subsequently marrying an American, was not considered by her parents to be entirely trustworthy when it came to carrying out this duty. It was for this reason that, every summer since she was three years old, Nadya had been shipped off for a month to her Mormor (her mother's mother) and Morfar (her mother's father). This year it was a family event. I was ready for a good vacation after a hard first year in Dumster. Taking that length of time off had presented a few problems at first, but after a little grumbling and a lot of negotiating, Dale Hurbalife agreed that he could cover my practice, so off we went.

Scandinavians have always fascinated me. They are so healthy. Every time I look at one of those tables that ranks the countries of the world according to some official measure of healthiness — like life expectancy or infant-mortality rate — Norway, Sweden, and Denmark are right up there one, two, three. Given the similarities between Vermont and Norway, I thought there might be some lessons in the Norwegians' life-style that I could bring back for the mutual edification of me and my patients. I decided to use this vacation to learn more about the habits of the people in this mysterious country.

All one has to do is look at a Norwegian to tell that he is healthy. His somber, expressionless demeanor contains not a hint of any of the frivolities of an ill-spent existence. How does he do it? What gives him the ability to thrive on adversity? Not wanting to omit anything that might have a bearing on the subject, I planned my investigation to include every facet of Norwegian life. I studied the weather (horrible). I studied the religion (Lutheran). I studied how they had a good time (don't). I examined how they buttoned their shirts (bottom to top) and how they ate their food (fork in the left hand).

One thing I learned pretty quickly: life in Norway is very different from life in the United States. Norway is a country where, when you leave your house to go for a stroll, and you meet someone coming in the other direction, that someone could just as well be a moose. It is a country where, when people get out snow tires for winter, they put them on their bicycles. It is a country where people pay very high taxes, but nobody complains about them. And it is a country where, when you go to the circus, and you get to the part where the pretty lady comes out in spangles and dances bareback while riding around the ring, the back on which she dances is that of a cow.

This is not to say that Norwegians lack imagination. On the contrary, it says that they have to do the best with what they have.

Another fact emerged as my studies progressed: the land of the midnight sun is a land of paradox. Take the midnight sun itself. It turns out that, just at the time of year when you need it most, it's nowhere to be found.

Norwegians are extremely proud of themselves, and with good reason. Despite this, the Bureau of Vital Statistics estimates that, at their current rate of reproduction, the only Norwegians left by the year 2400 will be Danes. This is not, I think, because Norwegians have a poor opinion of one another. It is more likely to be just an unfortunate complication of two Norwegian sleeping devices, the *sprekken* and the *dyne*. The *dyne* was invented by the Vikings, who had very poor central heating in their homes and very little female companionship. When a Viking went to bed, he would wrap his *dyne* around him like a cocoon. A *dyne*-covered Viking was as snug as a bug in a rug. This stood the Vikings in good stead for many centuries of long, hard winters. But as civilization came to the north country, and trees were gradually replaced by spouses and significant others, a problem arose. One *dyne* was not enough for two people, even under the most intimate circumstances. No big deal, said the Norwegians. We'll each have our own *dyne*. To prevent *dyne* poaching in the middle of the night, the Norskies introduced the *sprekken* to the conjugal bed. The *sprekken* is a narrow board that runs down the middle of a double bed. Made, symbolically, of wood, the *sprekken* ensures that each of the pair sticks to his or her own side and his or her own *dyne*. It does its job very well. (The Danes, who are more farsighted than the Norwegians, solved the *dyne* problem with an ingenious invention of their own, the double *dyne*. Consequently, while the Norwegians are fading into the woodwork, Danes are multiplying like bunny rabbits.)

Norway has fifteen types of pickled herring, but only one McDonald's, and no peanut butter.

Norwegians revere the sanctity of nature, but they consider Rudolph meat a delicacy.

Norway's favorite hero used to be Thor, a colorful fellow who rode around in a chariot drawn by two goats named Toothgnasher and Toothgrinder. He had a giant hammer that made thunder and lightning. He used the hammer for bashing ogres, trolls, and anybody he didn't like. With the arrival of Christianity, they abandoned Thor in favor of a guy named Martin, whose idea of having a good time was to put graffiti on church doors.

It was hopeless. The more I learned, the less I knew. Every point had a counterpoint. Every fact, an opposing one. After all my research, I still didn't feel I was any closer to the secret of Norwegian health. The night before we were to go back home, I confessed my failure to Arne and Knut.

"It's not something an American could understand," said Arne. "Unless you ate more fish."

"Too little fresh air," said Knut.

22

"*D* r. Conger?"
"Yes."

"This is Sarah. I'm sorry to bother you, but I have a question about one of your orders. I wonder if you could help me."

"I'd be glad to, Sarah. That's what doctors are for."

"It regards the patient you admitted today. Mr. Turmoller."

"What seems to be the problem?"

"Well, I wasn't sure if there was any particular time you wanted us to check his abdomen."

"I'm afraid I don't understand. Check his abdomen for what?"

"I'm sorry to be so stupid. When you wrote the order to mash on tummy every evening, you didn't say when. I just want to make sure that it was OK to do it after supper."

"Mash on tummy every evening?"

"Yes, Dr. Conger. That's what it says. At least it looks that way to me. Of course, I may have read it incorrectly."

"I don't see how that could happen. As it happens, I was just coming out to see how he was doing. We can review the orders when I get there."

"That would be very helpful."

I left the office and walked out to the nurses' station. Sarah was standing there with the order book in front of her. She showed me the entry in question. I looked at it. There was no doubt. "Mash on tummy every evening" was the most plausible interpretation of the words I had written.

"I suggest you check him at about six P.M."

"Very well. You know, Dr. Conger, you have such an imaginative way of expressing yourself. It makes reading your orders so interesting. At times — if you don't mind my saying so — I even find it entertaining. Oh. I almost forgot. Mr. Turmoller mentioned that his ulcer often acts up after meals, and he usually takes an antacid for it."

"I see. For his ulcer."

"Yes, for his ulcer. Maalox, I believe he said it was."

"Well, then, why don't we give him Maalox, one tablespoon after eating?"

"That sounds like an excellent idea. Shall I write it for you?" Sarah's voice had a slight catch to it as if she had something stuck in her throat.

"That would be fine."

"I'll take care of that right away. Thank you so much for coming out. It's much nicer to deal with silly little things like this in person."

"Yes. I quite agree. If that's all, I must be getting back to the office. Take care now."

"You too, Dr. Conger."

Exchanges of this sort between doctors and nurses are quite commonplace in hospitals. There are those who say that they occur because doctors have such poor handwriting that no one can understand them. These same people claim that the reason we write illegibly is because we think we are too important to take the time to write properly, because we are too arrogant to understand that we have a responsibility to express our intentions clearly, and because we are lazy to boot.

The people who say this are inconsiderate and callous. They are the kind of people who make a living out of being unsympathetic to doctors. People who haven't the faintest idea — and probably couldn't care less — as to the real reason we write the way we do.

It is because we are sensitive.

———————◄ ◆ ►———————

SERIOUS READER NOTE: Sensitive people have a great need to feel appreciated. They need to know that when they have something to say, the person to whom they are going to say it will be sympathetically inclined. They are therefore very cautious when it comes to expressing themselves, especially in writing. They don't go blabbing their thoughts down on paper for anyone to look at and possibly make fun of. They hide them a little — not so much that they are invisible; just enough to ensure they will be deciphered only by someone who is willing to take a little extra effort to understand what they mean . . . someone who is not likely to jump down their throats.

———————◄ ◆ ►———————

Being completely honest (which I always am, even though it hurts sometimes), I will say that sensitivity is not the only reason that doctors have such unique penmanship. Doctors, as one might expect from such special people, pride themselves on their individuality and creativity. It used to be that the practice of medicine offered more than ample opportunity for us to express these qualities. If a person went to ten doctors with the same complaint, he could count on getting ten different opinions, each one completely unrelated to the preceding, and each one a reflection of the personality of the physician offering it. But that has all changed. We have become faceless automatons mouthing identical words that we are programmed to utter, not because it is what we want to say, but because technology dictates that we must. Medicine could just as easily be rendered by a computer. Our individuality has been stifled.

Except when we write. When a doctor sets pen to paper, the traces he leaves behind are as much a part of him as his right arm.

Take Joel Shrank, our psychiatrist. Dr. Shrank, who is a master in Japanese calligraphy, has handwriting that can only be called a work of art. I can stare at it for hours. Everyone admires it so much that nobody minds having to ask him to translate it into English.

And Fred Cracker. Fred is a big, bold fellow, just the way a surgeon should be. But he writes in such teeny, tiny letters that it looks as if they were made by a mouse who stepped in an ink puddle and ran across the page. Fred does not do this to be difficult, but to make himself less intimidating to the staff. It is a very considerate gesture.

Or myself. I know how degrading it can be to a nurse's sense of professional self-esteem when a doctor comes in and writes an order and then says, "Do this and be quick about it." So I try to write my instructions in such a way as to give them not one but several possible interpretations. This gives the nurses a chance to decide for themselves what is best for the patient and then discuss it with me. It makes them feel useful. And it makes me feel wanted.

Which, after all, is what communication is all about.

23

*M*edical science has made spectacular advances in the past century. It was barely yesterday that our knowledge of what makes the body tick came from those whose imagination exceeded their intellect. Now, you can walk into a medical laboratory and find hormones being recreated, genes being redesigned, and babies being reproduced. You can step into a drugstore and buy a medicine that will kill the meanest of germs, strengthen the weakest of hearts, and grow hair on a billiard ball. You can stroll into an operating room and find old, worn-out organs being replaced with shiny new plastic ones. The litany of successes is endless. Well, almost endless. A few of Nature's tricks are still tucked safely up her sleeve.

What makes a head ache? We haven't the foggiest. How does the skin itch? Your guess is as good as ours. Why does the colon complain? Beats us.

Spastic colitis. Irritable colon. Gas. Call it what you will. The only thing we know for sure is that when the patient's intestines rumble, the doctor's pockets jingle. Why? Because they are so unpredictable, digestive disgruntlements often generate hasty visits to the doctor. Because there is no cure, the risk that any given visit will avert a subsequent one is negligible. And because there is no effective treatment, a physician can, in good conscience, order any number of tests and prescribe any number of drugs in order to get credit for the remission that invariably follows each flare-up.

One other observation about the colics rings the truth bell. People who worry tend to have similarly inclined intestines. Therefore, it should come as no surprise to learn that the colon of Fusswood was not only irritable, but at times could be downright obstreperous. I saw him two weeks ago for one such attack, the proximate cause of which was a comment by his wife that his two receding hairlines appeared to be merging into one.

I treated him with my favorite one-two punch: sawdust and Donnatal. The sawdust is full of fiber, and fiber is good for everything enteric, proof of which can be seen in the excellent health of beavers and termites, among whom diverticulitis and colon cancer are completely unknown. I prescribed Donnatal because it is one of those wonderful pills that contains a carefully formulated combination of drugs that are present in low enough concentrations as to be free of any effect whatsoever, be it good or ill.

Fusswood was back in for his obligatory follow-up. Its purpose was to give him an opportunity to congratulate me on my management of the case.

"How's the old tummy doing, Fuss?"

"The old tummy? Well . . . uh . . . not too bad. Er . . . great. Great! Yup. Just great. All better now."

Something was not right. Fusswood was not one to concede so easily to treatment of an illness.

"The Donnatal. Did you find it helpful?"

"Donnatal? Donnatal. The pills! They were fabulous, Doc. Best medicine you ever gave me."

"No problems with the dose schedule?"

"No trouble at all. Took 'em all. Just like the doctor

ordered. Hey. That's pretty funny, huh? Just like the doctor ordered."

"Quite. I seem to have forgotten to write it down. Perhaps you can refresh my memory. Just how did the doctor order them?"

"How? Well, One every . . . Uh. Meal. Meals! That's it. One pill after every meal. Yessir, my good old after-meal pill, I call it. Had one just after breakfast this morning. Slipped right down."

"That's funny. Usually I recommend taking them before meals. The pharmacist must have made a mistake. Do you have the bottle with you?"

"Er. No mistake, Doc. I take them before meals too. One before and one after. Figured I'd hit the old belly coming and going."

All this talk about pills seemed to make Fusswood restless. He got up from his chair and started to pace around the office. That's when I noticed it.

"Why, Fusswood. You're limping. Something the matter with your leg?"

"My leg? Naw. A little charley horse, that's all. Nothing for you to worry about, Doc. You're too busy."

This was most peculiar. Fusswood had never considered me too busy for any of his troubles. Something was quite wrong indeed.

"Fusswood, have you been seeing someone else?"

"Moi? After all you've done for me? Wouldn't dream of it." His pacing increased, and the limp became more noticeable.

"Fusswood!"

"It wasn't my fault, Doc. Honest. All I wanted was —"

"I warned you about this. If it's drugless treatment you want, it's drugless treatment you get. Now get lost. I've got too many loyal patients to waste my time on cheaters."

"Gimme a break, Doc. You told me it was OK if something happened to my back. Well, I wrenched it lugging in the wood. So I went over, and he took an X ray. It showed a couple of vertebrae out of place and a prolapsed colon too. He snapped my back in. Then he told me that to fix my colon, I would have to get rid of my pills, buy some new shoes, and come in for adjustments three times a week. What could I say? He's the doctor."

"He is *a* doctor, Fusswood. I am *the* doctor. And don't you forget it."

"You're right. It was a dumb thing to do. Still, after a couple of treatments, my bowels started to straighten out. You don't think that maybe . . . ?"

"Fusswood!"

"Sorry. Must be brain damaged from all that banging around. I promise it won't happen again. Just give me one more chance."

We of the healing professions are a forgiving lot. "All right. I'll let it go this time. Here's your prescription. Make an appointment for two weeks."

As a chagrined Fusswood hurried out the door, I got on the phone to J. Arthur Backslap, D.C.

There is little love lost between doctors of medicine and doctors of chiropractic. Nevertheless, since neither one has the medicinal arsenal to destroy the other without bringing himself down in the holocaust, we have learned to coexist. Like the Russians and the Americans, we defame each other in public and conduct our mutual business in private. Each leaves to the other that which is within his recognized sphere of influence. The aching back is behind the chiropractic curtain, but the complaining colon was mine. Backslap was poaching.

"Good to hear from you, Beachie. How's life among the dope pushers?"

"I just saw Fusswood. He came in here with your paw prints all over his colon. What's the story?"

"Hey, big fella. Don't get so touchy. How was I suppose to know it was yours? He didn't say anything, and I didn't see a No Trespassing sign on the X ray."

"Well, I'm telling you now, you manipulative creep. That bowel is posted. Prolapsed colon, my eye. I suppose it comes from eating too much spaghetti. Fortunately, I found out in time to avoid any permanent damage."

"I bet. Listen, while I got you on the phone, I wonder if we can change the time for our racquetball match on Thursday. It's a little late for me."

"I'd love to, Art, but it's out of the question. I get nervous playing when there are crowds around."

"So be it. I'll see you at three in the A.M."

"Nice shot, Beachie."

Match point. J. Arthur nervously swished his racquet back and forth as I raised mine for the serve.

Wham! It was a sizzling serve.

Plip. His feeble return floated harmlessly in front of me.

Whop! I smashed it back. As the winning point dropped untouched in the corner, I heard a snap, like someone stepping on a twig — but there were no twigs on the court.

Backslap ambled over. "Congratulations, big boy. Nice game. Hey, you OK?"

"Me? I'm fine. I always like to do a few minutes of stretching on the floor after a game. Keeps me limber. You go ahead. I'll join you in the locker room."

"Suit yourself." He turned to go. Then he looked back. "You sure there's nothing wrong?"

"Heavens, no! I'm in great shape." I wiggled my toes a few times as proof. Reassured, I attempted to rise. An electric shock ran up one leg, across my pelvis, and down the other. I collapsed in a pool of molten pain. Backslap was over me in a flash.

"I believe your back is out, old man. Here, let me fix it for you."

I lay there helpless, hurting, and humiliated. Four years of medical school. Four more of postgraduate training. Fifteen years of practice. And here I was at the mercy of a quack.

————◄ + ►————

SERIOUS READER NOTE: Doctors hold a pretty dim view of the science of chiropractic, which views the spine as a kind of skeletal woodpile, flimsily stacked and ready to tumble to the ground should one log happen to slip out of place. We, on the other hand, see it as a mighty rod, supple as birch and strong as steel. Flanked by thick sets of muscles and held together with more ligaments than I can ever remember, the back is capable of infinitely more self-adjustment than any pair of hands could effect. But the back is temperamental. It can withstand leaps from a tall building and crumble before a shoelace. And when it stops, it is not likely to start up again until it is good and ready, pushing and shoving notwithstanding. Not that spinal adjustments are completely useless: they can provide welcome relief for an aching back. But the idea of going to someone to have your back put in place every time it slips out makes about as much sense as going to the gas station after every rain to have your windshield wipers reset.

————◄ + ►————

None of this was the slightest consolation as I tried unsuccessfully to get up off the floor.

"Don't be such a stubborn fool, Mr. M.D. Lie still and let me fix you up. Don't worry. My lips are sealed. Besides, who would believe me?"

I had little choice. With a reluctant grunt, I rolled over and offered up my aching back. Backslap's sure hands quickly found the affected cranny. As he poked and probed, the pain began to melt away. I felt warm and tingly. It was nice. Very nice. J. Arthur knew his stuff.

"Hey, Art. Tell me the truth. You don't really believe all that hogwash about adjusting vertebrae, do you? I bet I could get the same service at a good massage parlor. And at half the price."

His hands moved suddenly. An excruciating pain shot into my neck and out my left ear.

"What the hell was that?"

"Sorry, big fella. Must've slipped. The old hands aren't what they used to be. You were asking my opinion about chiropractic theory. The scientific justification may be a little skimpy, but you've got to remember, chiropractic is only ninety years old. In the life of a healing art, we're just babes in the cradle. If I remember correctly, you guys spent about two thousand years pushing that four-humors stuff before Harvey figured out that blood traveled around in circles. And how long was it that your therapeutic guns were leeches, laxatives, and strychnine? I'll bet those patients felt great — when you stopped."

Backslap was right. The medical profession had perpetrated outright fraud on an unsuspecting public for centuries. It wasn't until the last fifty years that a patient had better than even odds at benefiting from a visit to his doctor.

He moved away and motioned for me to stand. "Give it a try, big boy."

I stood up — a little stiffly, but at least I could move.

"Thanks, Art. Hey. Not bad. I'd have to say the old column feels pretty well stacked. Maybe you got something there after all."

"Think nothing of it. Maybe you can return the favor someday and poison me with a few pills."

"Sure thing. Well, I gotta be going."

"Not so fast, fella. You're carrying around some major derangements on that overpaid skeleton of yours. This adjustment is just a finger in the dike. If you don't do something about it pretty soon, you could wind up a basket case. Let me set you up for a regular schedule of treatments. After hours, of course."

"Forget it. This is a one-shot deal. You guys really know how to milk the cow, don't you?"

"Listen, Beachie. If we only saw those patients who really needed our services, we'd both be on the breadlines in no time flat. You pack them in with your voice, I use my hands. What's the difference? If the fans like it, what's the harm?"

"No comprende, masher. But thanks for the service. Same time next week?"

"Your time is my time."

We parted in the predawn light, and I headed for my car. I opened the door, climbed in, and reached for the ignition. But it was too late.

The dike had burst.

24

*S*ince time immemorial, philosophers have debated the question "What is it about man that has made him foremost among the creatures who inhabit this earth?" In former times it was ascribed to favoritism on God's part. But today such a belief is considered unscientific and without merit. The possible answers to this question are many. Our ability to stand on two feet. The use of tools. Speech. But rigorous examination of the facts should make it clear that none of these is unique to *Homo sapiens*. A monkey can walk quite well. Beavers are master builders. And whales have a perfectly adequate language. But there is one quality of man that cannot be found anywhere within the animal kingdom — one that has given us the will to be the best. As the great muse once said, "To complain is human."

The poor pout about money. The rich rant about taxes. The industrious moan about fatigue, while the lazy languish over boredom. The fat fuss at the thin, and the skinny scowl at the plump. There is something wrong for everyone. This state of perpetual dissatisfaction with one's lot in life, this ability to see oneself as always worse off than his neighbor, is the one quality, more than any other, that has promoted advancement of the human race. Complaining has given us a collective lifting up by the other's bootstraps.

Even doctors complain. Given that they have been permitted to graze in the greenest of life's pastures, this accomplishment is no mean feat. But we are an imaginative and resourceful bunch. What is it that gets our goat? The long hours we work? The responsibility of holding another's life in our hands? Having to stare death in the face day after relentless day? None of these. It is a subject far more burdensome that clouds our countenances when we gather together in small groups, nodding and bobbing and looking grave. Malpractice. That is the fate we bemoan.

Malpractice. Drop the word in a medical pond and it lands like a boulder. Stir it into a doctor's soup and it sours the taste. Malpractice is the bitter pill, the screw that turns, the straw that breaks the camel's back. Any way you look at it, malpractice makes us sputter.

———— ◄ ✦ ► ————

SERIOUS READER NOTE: Why is malpractice the doctor's complaint? The reason is not what you might think. Cost? Premiums are indeed expensive, but they have no discernible effect on doctors' incomes, for they are paid not by us but by our patients. Inconvenience? The fuss and bother of a malpractice suit is handled by lawyers and insurance agents. Humiliation? By training and temperament we are constitutionally immune. Besides, every profession has these obstacles. But nobody else has malpractice troubles like the doctor. So the reason, plain and simple, that we wear malpractice as our millstone is that nobody else can.

———— ◄ ✦ ► ————

Yesterday morning, when I cruised into the cafeteria, there were Fred Cracker and Carl Cutterup in the doctors'

corner. (Emmeline Talbot was not big enough to have separate facilities for its doctors, but the corner served the
same purpose, since nobody else dared sit there, except
occasionally Mr. Shiftley or Sarah Trotter, and then only by
invitation.) I got a cup of tea and went over to join them.

"Pull up a chair," said Fred.

"Thanks, but I think I'll stand."

"Suit yourself," he replied, casting a glance at my awkward stance. "Back still giving you trouble? You've been laid
up with that for a month now. Those discs are mean babies.
You should let me fix it for you."

"My back is fine," I replied abruptly. "I'm just a little stiff
today."

"So I see. Say, why don't you go to Backslap. He'll
straighten you out, all right. Like a board." He chuckled
loudly at this witticism and returned to the topic that my
arrival had interrupted. "I can't believe it. Just got my notice from Neverslip. Did you see what our malpractice pre-
mium is going to be next year? Twenty-five thousand bucks!
That's outrageous. The way things are going, it doesn't pay
to get up in the morning."

"I know what you mean," concurred Dr. Cutterup. "If
Blue Cross hadn't just increased gallbladders to fifteen hundred per, I would have had to sell one of my Porsches."

"Yeah. But it isn't just the money. Look what it does to
our patients. Last week I had this guy in the office with a
bum hip. So, I tell him he needs a new one, which, I explain,
I am willing to give him. Then I tell him about the operation. You know what he said to me? 'Are you sure you have
told me all the risks?' I mean, if that doesn't take the cake.
I had half a mind to chuck him out on his ear."

"And the goddam lawyers," chimed in Dr. Cutterup.
"They're like vultures. No offense to your wife, Beachie,
but you know what I mean."

I nodded to indicate that I understood.

"Hey," said Fred. "Listen to this one. You know how to tell the difference between a dead skunk in the road and a lawyer? There's skid marks in front of the skunk."

Dr. Cutterup burst into laughter. I gave a polite titter. Dr. Cracker turned to me.

"This stuff doesn't bother you, does it, babe? With a lawyer for a wife, you've got your ass covered coming and going."

"Who would want to sue me?" I said deprecatingly. "I'm just a harmless pill pusher."

"Don't be so sure. The other day I read about a lady who collected one million bucks because her doctor said it was OK to take aspirin for her headache, and she came down with a goddam bleeding ulcer. Get this. The old dame had been taking six Anacin a day for twenty years, but the judge said that didn't matter because she didn't know it contained aspirin." He looked at his watch. "Well, boys, gotta go. You coming?"

"Where?"

"To the lecture on risk management. It's a tag-team job featuring Profetti and Philibuster. Should be good for laughs, anyway."

I had four patients in the hospital. I knew I should see them before office hours, but I didn't want to. They all had the same problem. No place to go. Too helpless to care for themselves, their spouses dead or similarly stricken, their children too busy, these unfortunate patients lay waiting in their beds, while each day nurses and social workers and therapists hovered over them in a futile effort to make the wait less a bother — futile not because they couldn't do anything, but because it wasn't really that much bother, since they, the waiters, had long since lost interest in the project. Patients who had only one thing left to do, and who dabbled at it now and then, but mostly waited, figuring that I could probably do it just as well for them as they could for themselves. And I could, for they were waiting to die. I decided they could wait for me until after the lecture.

To my surprise, most of the staff was there. Malpractice is like the weather. We talk about it a lot, but nobody ever does anything about it. Herbert Shiftley introduced the guests.

"I'm pleased to see so many of you here. I believe most of you know Joe Profetti from Neverslip Casualty and Insurance Company. And Theo here hardly needs an introduction. Mr. Profetti will start with a presentation on informed consent, after which Mr. Philibuster will discuss an exciting new concept in risk management. OK, Joe. Take it away."

"Thanks, Herb. Gentlemen. Er . . . gentlepeople. Sorry about that, Dr. Flushing. But you know how it is with old horses. You — "

"Make them into glue, I believe," interjected Dr. Flushing.

Joe laughed uneasily.

"Now where was I? Oh, yes. If you remember that patients are like children, it all falls into place. Tell a kid he can't go out when it's thirty below and snowing up a blizzard, and what happens? Whether or not the child will succeed in life, whether he will ever find happiness, whether, in fact, his life will have any meaning at all, immediately becomes solely dependent on his ability to commune with nature sometime in the next thirty seconds. But, inform that same child, on the very same day and at the identical hour, that he must go out to play, and a protest will arise that would make one think you had banished him from the face of the earth.

"Informed consent is no different. Should you begin by telling your patient that the issues involved in a particular therapeutic decision are too complex for him to grasp, he will demand that you recite the entire body of medical knowledge on the subject. But give him a little dose of unsolicited information, and before you can say 'Sign here,' you'll have him begging you to stop.

"Take a gallbladder operation, for example. Don't pussy-foot around. Tell him everything. Point out that a whiff of anesthesia might bust his cerebral thermostat and fry his brains right there on the table. Tell him about the pain and the insomnia and the risk of infection. Be sure to remind him that just when it looks as if he is out of the woods, his incision could split open, spill his guts all over the bed, and leave him with a scar the size of the Grand Canyon. Lay it on. The thicker the better. When you think your patient would rather be run over by a herd of stampeding buffalo than face the knife, play the flip side. Explain that whatever the risks might be for elective surgery, they are nothing compared to what might happen if you have to take out the gallbladder under emergency conditions. Tell them about the patient you had who was sitting in a restaurant enjoying her lobster Newburg, when she had an attack so sudden that it made her double over in pain. She struck her head on the table and hit her fork, which flew up in the air just as the waiter was coming by with a pot of hot coffee. The fork poked him in the eye, he spilled the coffee on her head, and she got a burn so bad that even after seventeen operations, her face has more potholes than Main Street in spring. Finish it all off with a discussion about the risk of cancer in gallbladders with stones. By the time you're done, he'll be eating out of your hand."

Profetti gave several more illustrative examples and sat down. Shiftley turned the meeting over to Theodore Quincy Philibuster, Esq.

"Too long have you physicians been forced to wage the malpractice war with one hand tied behind your back. Too long have you had to sit back and take blow after unrelenting blow from your ungrateful patients with no recourse but to turn the other cheek. Too long has the fight been fought on your soil. The time has come to change the course of battle. The time has come to unsheathe your swords. The time has come to attack. Forget about defensive medicine. Offensive medicine is your banner from here on out. In the words of Napoleon Bonaparte, 'The best defense is a good offense.' And what an offense you have at your disposal! Think about it. Why does a patient sue? Because he is unhappy. And why is he unhappy? Because he is dissatisfied. Get rid of his dissatisfaction and you can kiss your malpractice worries good-bye. How can you do this? Simple. You have in your possession a weapon that can level dissatisfaction with a single blow. Fear. That's all it takes. A frightened patient will never sue.

"I hardly need to tell such a distinguished collection of physicians how to instill terror in the hearts of your patients. But it might be instructive to show you how easy it is to turn a potentially litigious patient into one who is meek as a lamb. Here's how we'll do it. I'm going to take you through a hypothetical patient-doctor interaction that would take place when it is the patient who is on the defensive. Dr. Conger, you play the role of doctor. Dr. Flushing, perhaps you'd be kind enough to be a patient. And we'll need a nurse. How about you, Dr. Cutterup? Fine. Dr. Flushing, you're coming to see Dr. Conger about a lump under your arm. OK, folks, take it away."

"Dr. Conger, I'm so worried. I found thi —"

"Just a minute, Ms. Flushing," interrupted Philibuster. "Before you proceed with your complaint, I would like to inform you of your rights. You are suspected of having an illness. You have the right to remain silent. You have the right to an attorney. If you waive that right, anything you say may be used against you. Now, you may proceed."

"I have this lump, Doctor. It hurts terribly and I'm so worried about it. It could be something serious."

"Show me where —"

"I'm sorry, Ms. Flushing," interrupted Philibuster, "but I'm afraid Dr. Conger will not be able to treat you."

"Why not?"

"Doctor Conger does not take any cases which have the potential for turning into something serious."

"Oh. Then I guess he'll have to refer me to someone who does."

"That's quite out of the question," said Philibuster. "Dr. Conger does not make referrals. The potential liability is too great. Should you experience a therapeutic misadventure, an undue complication, or an unforeseen outcome while under the care of another physician, such care being the result, directly or indirectly, of a recommendation by Dr. Conger, or should you incur an injury on the way to said physician, it could be construed, as a result of such recommendation, that Dr. Conger, his heirs and assigns, would all be negligent per se and accordingly held liable for any adverse consequences resulting from such misadventure, complication, or outcome."

"But I have to do something. This is very painful."

I looked at Philibuster. He shook his head. "I'm sorry," I said. "There's nothing I can do."

"Please understand, Ms. Flushing," said Philibuster. "The last statement of Dr. Conger is merely an expression of his personal feelings. In no way should it be considered a professional opinion. Nor should any of the aforeto mentioned statements be construed as a refusal to provide treatment. Dr. Conger is perfectly willing to treat you for any condition which is pursuant to the nature of his practice."

"What good does that do me?"

"Well," I said, trying to be helpful, "maybe there is something else bothering you that I could take a whack at."

"Only my back. But that always gives me trouble when I've been putting in extra hours at work."

"Back is out," said Philibuster.

"That's what I thought. But I went to Dr. Backslap, and he said it was OK."

"I am not referring to the state of your back, Ms. Flushing. I am referring to Dr. Conger's ability to treat you. He does not accept any cases which could involve litigation or workmen's compensation. I suggest you try again."

"That's all I got — except a sore throat I had last week. But it's fine now."

"That sounds highly suitable." Philibuster beamed, turning to me. "OK, Doc. Do your thing, Doc."

"A sore throat, you say. Did you happen to have any other symptoms with it? Like a fever or perhaps a cough?"

"Yes. I had a high fever for several days."

"What was your temperature?"

"I don't know, but my husband said I felt like a boiled lobster."

"I'll have to object to that last statement, Ms. Flushing," said Philibuster. "An out-of-office statement by a third party, to wit, your husband, rendered for the truth of the matter, is hearsay. Without a verified thermometer reading, Dr. Conger will have to consider your allegations regarding the fever as inadmissible."

"I had a headache too."

I looked at Philibuster. He nodded. "Headache can be an important symptom," I said, beginning to get the hang of things. "It will require a thorough investigation. In addition to a blood count, mono spot, AIDS test, throat culture, and urinalysis, you'll need a chest X ray, spinal tap, CT scan of the brain, gallbladder ultrasound, and a pregnancy test."

"A pregnancy test for a sore throat?"

"Dr. Conger is just making sure he doesn't overlook anything," replied Philibuster. "If you do not wish to comply with his recommendations, that, of course, is your prerogative. But I must ask you to sign this waiver of liability for refusal to follow medical advice in order to absolve Dr.

Conger of any consequences that might accrue pursuant to said refusal." He passed her a sheet of paper. "Mr. Cutterup, would you be so kind as to witness Ms. Flushing's signature?"

"Don't bother."

"I beg your pardon?"

"I said, 'Don't bother.' I'm not signing anything. I came in here for a serious medical problem, which you refuse even to look at. Then I tell you about something that I don't even have anymore, and you want to put me through a thousand dollars' worth of tests. I never heard anything so ridiculous in all my life. I'm getting out of here." She wadded up the paper and threw it in Philibuster's face.

"Excuse me, please," said Philibuster. "Mr. Cutterup, did you hear Ms. Flushing's last statement? Very good. Well then, that should do it. Thank you very much, Ms. Flushing. You've been most helpful. Dr. Conger will be in touch with you."

"Oh no, he won't," cried Liz. "I'm not coming back here again!"

"We are not referring to seeing you here. The remarks you have just made regarding Dr. Conger's professional abilities constitute a flagrant defamation of character. Dr. Conger will see you in court."

25

Dear Chip,

Good news! I'm finally going to be able to break away from things here in Pleasantville to come up for the long-awaited visit. It hardly seems possible that it's really going to happen after all these false starts, but it's true. I've got tickets to arrive on the 6 PM bus Friday. Can't wait to see your new home. And your hospital!

Hope your back is better. See you soon.

Love,
Mom

*I*t had finally come. Mom's first visit to Dumster. It was no coincidence that there had been so many "false starts." For over a year I had managed to procrastinate and prevaricate my way out of each of a half-dozen threatened landings, but now the stalling was over. Mom was coming to Dumster.

I am a good son. I call home on Sunday night, and I try to get down to Pleasantville every couple of months to pay my respects. Trine is a dutiful daughter-in-law. She listens politely to Mom's suggestions for self-improvement and agrees enthusiastically when I suggest we take her with us on vacations. Being with Mom is not the problem. Mom coming to Dumster is.

When my mother decided that it would be a good thing for me to become a doctor, this was no casual fancy on her part. She had had extensive experience with her Uncle Ned, and although she never worshipped him as Aunt Helen did, she recognized his value in advancing the family honor. She was especially cognizant of the respect his mother got as the person who was responsible for producing such a wonderful doctor. When I was in medical school, she often talked about what it would be like when I had my own practice: adoring patients, devoted nurses — a son who was beloved and respected by all.

I didn't turn out to be the doctor my mother expected. I have not become the kind of distinguished, dignified person a doctor ought to be. Although outwardly I am treated with the utmost respect, I can tell that behind the "Yes, Dr. Conger" and "Whatever you say, Dr. Conger," people are secretly laughing at me. I can tell because I am a sensitive person. A sensitive person is extremely aware of his appearance — more aware even than those who look at him. A sensitive person can see in himself blemishes and absurdities that a casual observer would overlook completely. A sensitive person knows that he looks ridiculous even when others don't know it. This means that if a sensitive person is a doctor, he cannot wear a white coat.

Snakes. Liver. Needles. Everybody has one. An object, perfectly harmless to others, for which they would rather go through fire and brimstone than to experience. Mine is a white coat.

I have donned a white coat only once in my medical career. I was a second-year medical student. It was my first day of physical diagnosis at Boston City Hospital. Each of us received a slip of paper on which was written the name of the patient we were to examine and the ward on which the patient was located. Our instructor explained that our assignment for the first day was to find the patient and then return within the allotted time to his office. That would be challenge enough, he explained upon seeing the disappointed looks on our faces. "Muriel Reilly. Peabody 2" read my card.

"Nurse!"
"Shut up!"
"Doctor!"
"Shut up!"
"Help me!"
"Shut up!"

A light snow fell through a broken window in the glass ceiling. In the dull yellow light that barely illuminated the ward, I could make out two rows of beds lined up against each of the long walls and separated one from another by thin curtains. In one of them an indistinct figure appeared to be struggling. The exchange between this figure and some invisible being in another of the beds was apparently occasioned by my arrival on the ward, there being no other signs of ambulatory life in the vicinity. Desperately I looked around for some more authoritative figure to relieve me. But I was alone. Stimulated by the dialogue, the other patients chimed in until soon a cacophony of cries reverberated throughout the room, transforming it from a hospital ward to an aviary. I tore off my coat and threw it on the floor. As suddenly as it had begun, the noise stopped. Forgetting my nascent professional dignity, I fled the scene and retreated to the safety of my instructor's office.

* * *

I have managed to hide my failing for twenty-three years. I did my training in city hospitals, where dignity is a handicap, not an asset. Then I went to Berkeley, where it is irrelevant. And now to Dumster, where people, although they know I am a misfit, don't throw it up at me. Because Dumsterians are a tolerant lot. The people who live here were either born here, in which case they don't know how the rest of the world functions, or they moved here from somewhere else because they do know and can't do it. In the words of that great Vermont poet, "If you have to come here, they have to take you in." Which is why it's been the perfect place for us. Well, almost perfect. Trine has had some difficulty finding her space. She didn't say much when we first moved here, and people started calling her Congers, but when she discovered it was her middle name — the first being Doctor and the last being Wife and all three pronounced as a single word, Doctorcongerswife — she pretty near exploded. However, with a little good nature and a lot of patience, she's managed to accept Dumster's inability to recognize that she is her own person, because putting up with me has sufficient redeeming value to grant tolerance of this shortcoming.

"Let's go to the hospital," Mom said as soon as I had gotten her bags into the car.

"Why don't we go home first? The kids are dying to see you."

"The kids can wait. I want to see my son's castle."

It was no use trying to talk her out of it. Besides, I had to face the music sometime; it might as well be now.

We pulled into the parking lot. "Well, Mom, this is it."

"Oooh. It's lovely. Just as I imagined it. Where's your office?"

"It's the one in the corner."

"You must have such a view."

"I do, Mom, a great view."

"Well, we'll come back to the office tomorrow. Now, I want to see the hospital."

"This is it, Mom."

"Come now, Chip. You can't be too tired to show me the hospital. You said it wasn't far away from your office."

"It isn't, Mom."

"Well, let's go then."

"There's no place to go. This is the hospital."

"And I am the Queen of England. All right, let's go see the hospital." Mom hopped out of the car and marched in the main entrance. By the time I caught up with her she had discovered the truth.

"Well, I guess the joke's on me." Forcing a smile, she slipped her arm through mine. "Well, My Son, the Doctor, lead the way."

We had gone about halfway down the corridor when Mom stopped. "We can't go to see your patients looking like this."

"Don't worry, Mom. You look fine. Besides, you're with me."

"That's what I mean."

"I think they'll recognize me even with a good-looking woman on my arm."

"Your coat?"

"My coat? It's in the car. That way I won't forget it. You see, Mom, I'm responsible now."

"Your white coat."

"Oh. That coat. Well . . . I . . . uh, I'll get it. Don't move."

I left my mother standing in the hall while I went to the doctors' offices. Carl Cutterup always wore a white coat, and he was about my size. As luck would have it, he was not in, and there, hanging from its hook, was a freshly starched clean white coat. I took it off the hook. Suppressing the shiver that ran down my spine as I slipped my arm into one sleeve, I threw it on and headed back. At the door I met Liz Flushing.

"Well, don't we look like the well-dressed physician today," she joked. "Trying out a new image?"

"Oh, no. Just spilled some coffee on my shirt."

"All I can say, fella, is it's you."

I hurried back to Mom. She was ecstatic. "You look wonderful, son. Just the way I imagined."

We entered the nurses' station. The small talk stopped as soon as they saw me.

I introduced Mom. "Mother, this is Sarah Trotter, our head nurse, Karen Turgeon, and Tom Puffin, our respiratory therapist. Folks, this is my mother."

"Pleased to meet you," said Mom.

"The pleasure is ours, Mrs. Conger," said Sarah.

"Well, how are my patients today, Sarah?"

"Very well, as always, Dr. Conger."

"Is there anything they need?"

"Nothing at all, Dr. Conger. Everything is in order."

"I'm just going to show my mother around a bit."

"That sounds very nice, Dr. Conger. If you need me for anything, just call."

"I don't think that will be necessary, Sarah, but thank you for offering."

"My pleasure, Dr. Conger, sir."

I couldn't help noticing the new respect with which I was being treated. Was it my mother? Or was it my attire? Maybe I had been wrong about white coats all these years. I resolved to pick up some for myself first thing next week.

After I had shown Mom around, we came back to the nurses' station.

"Well, that takes care of the grand tour. I think we'll be heading home now."

"Good-bye, Dr. Conger. Thank you ever so much for bringing your mother around." She turned to Mom. "You have no idea how honored we are to meet you, Mrs. Conger. It's not every hospital that has a doctor like your son."

Mom nodded to acknowledge the compliment, and we left. As we headed back down the corridor, a muffled noise came from the nurses' station. It was the sound of voices. Not talking voices; voices that seemed to be — But they couldn't. Not in Dumster.

❧ 26 ❧

It was the slippers that reminded me.

I thought I had forgotten her. Purged her life from my files. Erased her death from my memory. Then one day a nurse pulled out the big cardboard box that held all the unclaimed clothes of those patients whose hospital exit was such that no one noticed a few missing items of apparel, and out fell a heavily worn pair of purple slippers. Her slippers.

The nurses called her Belle after the bell she brought with her whenever she came to the hospital. She preferred it to the bedside call button, which blended so harmoniously with the other instruments in the hospital orchestra that when struck, it was barely noticeable. Belle's bell was metal with a push button on top — the kind that, if you know how to play it, could sound like a cymbal. Belle was a virtuosa on her bell. When she rang, it rang for all to hear. And woe betide the poor soul who tarried in harking to its call.

Edward Francis Xavier McCue was a red-faced Irishman who for thirty years was Dumster's chief of police. He retired rather unexpectedly after forgetting to put on the emergency brake in his cruiser before jacking it up to change a tire. Until that time, Catherine had been his wife. Now she was his widow. In truth, it was Edward Francis

Xavier who was the husband of Belle, but it seems only fitting to give him a recognition in death that he never achieved in life — that of having an existence in his own right. For when Catherine Elizabeth Conley, at the age of sixteen, stood up at the altar and agreed to take his name, she did exactly that, and from that day hence, the former Edward Francis Xavier McCue became McCue's Old Man.

People said that Eddie drank too much. Those who knew them both said he didn't drink enough. McCue, she called herself, shunning her first name, not so much because it was a sign of femininity or friendliness, neither of which anyone had ever accused her of, but because it hinted of soft. McCue hated softness. She had raised seven children without any help from her husband, worked full-time to supplement Eddie's income, most of which dissolved in alcohol, and, on those not infrequent occasions when her husband was too drunk to perform his duties, run the police department. Family and work alike she ran without mercy, favoring intimidation over persuasion and invective over compassion. It was not the kind of treatment that fostered love, but it did get results. Each of her children was well behaved and well educated, and each, upon reaching the age of maturity, left Dumster never to return again.

McCue was eighty-seven when I met her. It was a mystery to everyone how she had achieved this inordinate longevity. But one thing was clear: it was not the result of walking the straight and narrow. McCue drank almost as much as her husband, and her bony fingers were only without a cigarette when one was dangling between her lips. It was no mystery to McCue. When I asked her why she had lived so long, she replied, "The Lord don't want me, and the devil won't take me." Father O'Shea, who was our local expert on such matters, concurred with her opinion.

But that wasn't the real reason. What kept her alive was her stubbornness. McCue was the most obstinate person I have ever laid hands on. Nobody ever convinced her of anything, and certainly no one ever got her to change her ways, except when she did it to prove she was right. Whenever I suggested some treatment for her ailments, which were legion, she either refused on the grounds that it would only make things worse, or agreed and promptly fell ill. She totally stripped me of any remaining illusion that medicine was a healing profession. She even made me consider quitting. But I didn't, if for no other reason than to prevent her from having the satisfaction of knowing she was more stubborn than I. Which she was.

McCue was the second patient I saw on my first day of work in Dumster. She wanted to waste no time checking out her new adversary.

"Let's get a few things straight, young man. At least 'man' is what you ought to be for all the papers you got hanging on the wall, but to look at you I would say you was hardly weaned. It took me most of twenty years to train Franklin. I haven't got that kind of time to waste on you. So you better listen good. You probably think that just because you can take a poor soul's last few pennies and make her sick as a dog (which, if she had really wanted to be, she could have stayed home and done for free), you're God's gift to the world. Let me tell you something. You ain't. You're no damn good. None of you. You barely listen. You hardly care. And you never think. Why every last Jack one of you ain't been arrested for murder and locked up I don't know, and I don't care. But you ain't going to do it to me. So, if you want to doctor on me you gotta know three things. First, don't give me no pill you ain't tried yourself. Second, no yapping. None of this 'We could do this. Or we could do that. It's up to you' malarky. It ain't up to me, and we both know it. Besides, you're all such a damn bunch of liars anyway, I'd never know the truth. Just do what you gotta and be quiet about it. Third, don't you ever slack up on me.

I'm an old bag — no point in pretending otherwise. But that doesn't mean I'm ready to kick the bucket. You give me your best or you give me nothing. OK, here's my pills." She pulled out of her pocketbook a plastic bag containing a dozen or so small bottles and threw them on my lap. "They're all poison." With the same gesture, she slipped out of her dress. "And here's my body. It looks like shit, but it's the only one I got. So be careful with it." She punctuated her last admonition with a dry cough and dragged her naked body up onto the table. "Now get to work."

It was all I could do not to gasp at the sight of her. Age had conspired with disease to strip her tiny body down to the bare bones, each one of which was distinctly outlined by the thin skin that was stretched tightly over it as if not quite enough had been allocated for the purpose. In a few spots it had worn out, and the underlying bone lay exposed to the outside world. Every blood vessel stood out in sharp relief. Calcified arteries bounded tumultuously against their restraints, and serpentine veins crossed the surface like tributaries of a river. Her spine, long since depleted of calcium, was so crooked that her line of vision was restricted to an area about six inches in front of her feet. Which was just as well, for that was as far as she could see through her cataracts.

She gasped for a few minutes from her effort and lay back on the table. Then she coughed. It was an incredible cough. If I hadn't heard it myself, I wouldn't have believed that her fragile body could produce something of such magnitude. Where she got the strength I have no idea, but it shook her delicate frame so violently that I feared the whole thing would collapse under its force.

"What seems to be the trouble today, Mrs. McCue?" I asked. The question was absurd, but under the circumstances it was the best I could do.

"Jesus, Mary, and Joseph!" she exclaimed. "How did I get

stuck with you? Are you blind, or just stupid? What the hell do you think is wrong? I'm dying. If" — a paroxysm of coughing temporarily interrupted her diatribe — "all you're going to do is gawk and yap, I'm leaving. By the way, it's McCue. No goddam Missus about it. Only damn thing I ever got from that good-for-nothing — God rest his soul — husband of mine." She finished up this brief eulogy by hastily crossing herself and then collapsed in a heap, exhausted by the effort.

I couldn't argue with her assessment. Her frail body drooped, like a heavily decorated Christmas tree, under the weight of the ornaments that adorned it. Heart failure. Ulcers. Arthritis. Cataracts. Emphysema — especially emphysema. Her lungs could barely move enough air to light the perpetual cigarette, and even that was a trial, so that she had to rest between each puff to catch her breath. How she managed to speak, let alone with such vehemence, escaped me completely.

She was a Pandora's box of pathology. An internist's delight. I set to work with a vengeance and gave her a going-over the likes of which Doc Franklin never dreamed of. By the time I was done recording my inspections and explorations, a person reading her record would have had trouble recognizing that my entry belonged in the same chart as its immediate predecessor, which read:

Feels lousy. Looks worse.
Two Green Pills

I summarized it all to McCue just as she had requested. "You are underfed and overmedicated. You smoke too much, and you exercise too little. Your lungs are rot. Your heart is shot. Your gut is gone. You are right. You should be dead."

"Talk is cheap," she replied. "What are you going to do about it?"

"Me, nothing. You, plenty. Throw away your pills. Stop smoking. Get a hot meal delivered at dinner. And walk ten minutes every day."

McCue rolled her eyes. "Mother of God! He's trying to kill me."

To prove her case, she followed my instructions to the letter. Her brain, in celebration of its drug-free existence, went into convulsions. I had to put her to sleep for two days with sodium pentothal. Without cigarettes, her normally dour unpleasantness was elevated to such heights that she got arrested. Twice: once for assaulting the postman with her cane after he delivered a letter from her daughter; then for creating a public nuisance, when she threw a tuna sandwich at Nat because it had too much mayonnaise. On my well-balanced diet, she lost five pounds. She had just recovered from the last of these setbacks when I reminded her about the walking. "You'll be sorry," she said. Her first time out, she tripped on the curb and broke four ribs. When she arrived in the emergency room, she was blue as a berry and barely conscious. She had two collapsed lungs and no discernible blood pressure. I told her the only hope was to put her on a respirator. She told me to call Father O'Shea. I agreed to do the one if she allowed the other. After two months in the ICU with mechanical breathing, intravenous feeding, and daily last rites, she was no better, but she was no worse — which was good, since the only thing worse was dead.

The only person who came to visit her was Father O'Shea. Sometimes her children called to see if she was still alive. I told one of her daughters that this might be a time to attempt reconciliation. She suggested that I ask McCue.

"The hell with 'em," said McCue. I decided to take matters into my own hands. On Mother's Day I sent her some flowers and signed them "Love, Carolyn." She saw through it and refused to speak to me for a week.

But during the third month of her hospitalization, a change came over McCue. Sarah noticed it first when she observed that McCue no longer rang her bell at every change of shift, the time she knew to be most difficult for nurses to answer her call. I wouldn't say she became anything like pleasant. She still complained about everything we did for her and anything we didn't, but not with the same gusto, as if her heart were no longer in it. One day she let a nurse feed her. On another she let one give her a back rub. Before we realized what had happened, McCue had actually become tame. The snarling cur who had landed on our doorstep was not exactly a docile little lap dog, but at least she could be touched without fear of being bitten. She never admitted as much, of course, but there could be no doubt. She liked it. For the first time in her life McCue was being spoiled, and it definitely suited her. The nurses, warming to the task, doubled their efforts. She became a pet. McCue rallied. She got off the respirator, and she started to eat. We had to do everything for her. Feed her. Bathe her. Empty her bowels and bladder. Even light her cigarettes. On her one hundred and thirtieth day in the hospital she took her first steps. Two people had to hold her up, but nonetheless, she was on the move. I decided she was ready for some real rehabilitation. I sent her across the hall to our rehabilitation unit, where she could get more intensive therapy. McCue hated it. Spoiling, she conceded, was something she could put up with. But therapy was another matter.

"Torture with a fancy name," she said. "That's all it is. I ain't going to be pestered to death. Send me home."

I said she couldn't possibly make it, but McCue was adamant. "Worst can happen is I die, and that ain't so bad, is it?"

We had a big celebration on her day of discharge, including live music and a lobster and champagne dinner. She gave the meal her supreme compliment: she ate it in silence. Then I dressed up in a red wig and played a song on my banjo. She smiled once in the middle and cried at the end. It was a silly song sung more or less to the tune of "Red River Valley." It went like this:

ODE TO McCUE ON HER LEAVING

From our hospital you will be going.
We will miss your sweet cough and kind word.
But we've ridded you of pseudomonas,
And your lungs are the clearest I've heard.

Come and take all your pills if you love me,
And your iron and vitamins too.
And remember the wonderful nurses,
And the Doc who has loved you so true.

I remember those times in ICU,
When your spirits had sunken so low.
And you called for the Good Lord to take you,
And she said, "All booked up. Try below."

So you tried out your luck with the devil,
And he came with a ring from your bell.
But when asked if he had any room there,
He said, "Belle, you've got no place in Hell."

So we trundled you over to rehab,
Where we tried to teach you how to dress
And behave like a right proper lady,
Which put you in a mighty distress.

I'll admit I thought you would not make it.
I was sure you would never get out.
I don't know what I'll do when you're gone, Belle.
I guess I'll just sit here and pout.

I didn't have to pout for long. Seven o'clock the next morning, she was back on our doorstep.

"What happened, McCue?" I asked.

"I got lonely."

I put her back to bed and reordered the same medicines. That night I was awakened at two in the morning by a call from the nurse. Belle had just told her that she was dying and that if I wanted to say good-bye, I should get in there pretty quick. I asked the nurse if she looked any different. She said no, she seemed comfortable, and her vital signs were stable. This being routine behavior for McCue, I told the nurse to tell her I'd be there first thing in the morning. When I got there next morning, I visited with her briefly. Then I signed her death certificate.

I think she did it on purpose. To prove once again that she was right. So that I wouldn't forget who was the boss after all those months the two of us were fighting tooth and nail over who was going to be in charge of her body. And so that I wouldn't forget what she had kept saying each time we argued over her health. "I'm dying, I tell you. 'Cause I sure ain't living. And if you ain't living, you're dying."

She wasn't really. Dying, that is. She was living — living just so she could show what it was all about to a whipper-snapper who thought he was keeping her alive with his medicine, when he was actually doing it with ignorance. And who never said good-bye or thank you.

Until now.

⚓ 27 ⚓

G *randma Canfield* is a remarkable person. She is ninety
years old and lives by herself in the family home in
Kokomo. She smokes a pipe, drinks a shot of brandy every
morning, and never goes to the doctor. But this is not why she
is remarkable. Grandma Canfield is the world's greatest ac-
cumulator. She has never thrown away anything. I don't
mean she literally hasn't thrown anything away: Grandma
Canfield is not a garbage collector. But she hangs on to all
that stuff people keep because they think someday it might
be useful, or if not actually useful, at least the source of
pleasant memories; stuff that, when they get a little further
down the line on the streetcar of life, people realize is starting
to get a little too cumbersome, so they leave it off at the next
stop. Grandma Canfield doesn't. She has her first jump rope
and the washboard she bought when she was married in 1910
and the stubs to every show she has ever seen and every
Christmas present she has been given by her five children,
thirteen grandchildren, and twenty-five great-grand-
children. If anyone were to ask Grandma Canfield why she
kept all this stuff — which, to the best of my knowledge, no
one ever has — she would probably tell them this: "Someone
cared enough to give 'em to me. Least I can do is keep 'em."

Last week a man came into my office who reminded me of Grandma Canfield. His name was Anatoli Pakhrat. He cherished pills the way she revered memorabilia. Mr. Pakhrat was the director of a movie they were making in Dumster. The movie had caused quite a stir in town. Dumster wasn't used to much attention in the tourist way, and all of a sudden there were hundreds running around. People were on their best behavior. Including me. The movie folk were different from Dumster patients. They don't have time for things like being sick. And they have this feeling, which I think comes from working with illusions so much, that the course of an illness can be altered by going to the doctor. They're not much for tincture of time.

Anatoli Pakhrat looked awful. Even the cat would think twice before dragging him in. His skin was the color of dishwater, and beads of perspiration clung to its surface like a swarm of insects. Great bags of eyelids hung from his brow, which was so contorted in its largely futile effort to maintain a line of vision that his features were barely recognizable. In the middle of his face was a huge red appendage. From its location, there could be no doubt as to what it was, but in its current state, the red, turgid object bore a much closer resemblance to an organ of the lower regions than it did to a facial one. This likeness was strengthened by the intermittent emission from its orifices of a thick, milky discharge.

"I'b dyig," he said after I inquired as to the nature of his problem.

"Quite true, Mr. Pakhrat. As are we all. In your case I would estimate about forty years, barring the unforeseen, of course."

"I got a ruddy node," snuffled Anatoli.

I looked up the old proboscis. "You're absolutely right."

"Ad a sore throat."

Into the mouth I peered. "Right again."

"Ad a cough," mustering as evidence a feeble hack.

"Three for three. Sir, your diagnostic acumen astounds me. You should have been a doctor."

"Dot edough modey," scoffed Anatoli. "I thig I got tribble dubodia, ad baybe sidus too."

"You have a cold."

"Ibossible. I take two thousad billigrabs of vitabid C every day."

"Vitamin C won't keep you from getting a cold."

"But Lidus Paulig said — "

"Linus Pauling was a great quantum chemist, but he didn't know vitamins from neutrinos. Vitamin C won't keep you from getting a cold. And in your case I would say that's quite fortunate."

"You're glad I have a code?"

"Most definitely. I would say you got it just in the nick of time. At the pace you've been working. I would have predicted total collapse of the system in about two weeks. Now you're home free."

"But I'b sig!"

SERIOUS READER NOTE: Anatoli, like most people, was operating under the misconception that, simply because it is caused by a germ, a cold is bad for you. Nothing could be further from the truth. Most germs are friendly, helpful creatures. It is germs in the ground that decompose our waste products so the world does not become a giant garbage heap. It is germs in our intestines that allow us to digest the food we eat. It is germs in our nose and throat that stand guard over our body portals to protect us from the hostile advances of those few warlike relatives who have given the clan an undeservedly bad name. And it is germs in the laboratory, harnessed and domesticated, that work hard day and night designing more nutritious foods and making lifesaving medicines. We would be in real trouble without germs.

Including cold germs. In the battle of life, colds are firmly allied with the forces of good. A cold is man's best friend.

"That can't be true!" my patients say when I explain all this. Their brains have been addled by too much vitamin C and their power of reason clouded by propaganda from the drug manufacturers. "How can something that makes my eyes droop, my nose run, and my body crawl be good for me?"

It is true that a person with a cold looks quite sick — much sicker, in fact, than he actually is. This allows him all the benefits of a serious illness but none of the risk. He can eat whatever he wants ("Stuff a cold and starve a fever."), sleep to his heart's content ("Get plenty of rest."), and even kiss his responsibilities good-bye ("We'll take care of it.").

But these are only the fringe benefits of a cold. A cold's real value is that it gets you sympathy. Sympathy is very important to people. Unfortunately, sympathy is one of those things that, the more you try to get it, the more elusive it becomes. A person who goes around saying 'Poor me' all the time is sure to be told that life is tough and be summarily dismissed. But let that same person come down with a case of the sniffles, and it will be a different tune altogether.

Serious readers by now are no doubt beginning to see a cold in its true light. And you may be saying to yourselves, "How can I get a cold when I need one?" This is easy. First you must find a cold virus. If you are a doctor, a teacher, or a parent, it's no problem. The cold will come to you. Should you not be so fortunate, the best thing to do is shake hands with everyone you meet. Colds are transmitted most effectively by hand-to-hand contact.

Once you have acquired the virus, it must be incubated. Cold air is not all that helpful, but dry air is very beneficial. The surest way to guarantee the right environment for the hatching of your cold is to keep your mouth open. (Although other reasons have been of-fered, it is likely that this proclivity of the cold virus explains why so many politicians have red noses.)

"Doe good," said Anatoli when I had finished my explanation. "Eberybody out there is as sig as I ab."

"That complicates matters. If colds are to serve their purpose, it is very important that they not be contracted simultaneously by all members of a sympathy-exchanging group."

"So ged rid of it."

"That could be difficult. You see, I've seen a lot of colds, even had a few myself, but I've never actually treated one. It's not one of the things we country docs are trained for. I wouldn't know where to begin. But, say, you seem to know a lot of medicine. What would you suggest?"

"Pills!"

"Pills. An excellent idea. How about Dripstop? It's a great decongestant."

"Dobe."

"Is there some reason you can't take it?"

"Already hab."

"Hmmm. Maybe we ought to give you some antibiotics. It won't do much for the cold, but should you get bronchitis or sinus trouble, they could be a real boon. Amoxicillin is my favorite, but we could use either erythromycin or Vibramycin if you prefer."

"Too late."

"You're taking all three?"

"Yup. Got Aboxicillid in Califordia, erythro in Rio, ad I always take wod Vibratab a day — they say it keebs the doctor away."

"Guess they said wrong."

"Yeah. Baybe I should boost it to two."

"Let's see. You're already taking antibiotics and decongestants. That doesn't leave much . . . Motrin! That's what you need. It's a great anti-inflammatory drug. Should make you feel like a million bucks."

"What do you tage be for? Sob bozo just off the traid? I've beed droppig Big Eb's siss they cabe od the barket. Keeps the old joids lubed. Forget the kids' stuff. I deed sobethig strog."

"Gee, that doesn't leave much else, except — But you wouldn't like it."

"I deber bet a drug I did't like."

"It's pretty strong stuff. Most of the people who took it have died."

"What's it called?"

"Can't tell you. Don't want it to get in the wrong hands. City people. You know how they are with drugs. Not that I would expect you to, but I got to play it safe. Anyway, I'll give you a couple."

"Two pills? That's all?"

"I told you this was powerful stuff. Here." I handed him the small brown envelope that I'd put in my drawer almost fifteen months ago after I had treated Aaron Penstock for his back. Several times I had pulled it out to try on a particularly difficult case, but each time I had lost my nerve. This time, I was determined to see it through. Besides, I had nothing to lose. Anatoli would never tell. "Take them now. Then go straight home, lie down, and stay in bed for four hours. When you get up, you should be cured. If you aren't, call me immediately. I'll have to ship you out to Boston tonight."

"OK, here goes dothig." Anatoli swallowed the two Green Pills.

"Good. Now remember. Four hours on the dot."

"Take four. Righto."

Four hours later Maggie came in to tell me that a Mr. Pakhrat was on the line. "I told him you were busy, but he insisted. He said you told him to call."

"I'll take it, Maggie. I should have known better."

"I'm afraid I don't understand."

"Never mind. I just tried a treatment I had no business using. Put him through."

"Doc. Adatol Pakhrat here. I gave it four hours. Just lige you said. You dow what your pills did? Dothig! Big zero. I got reservashuds od the five o'clock plade to Bostid. Dice try, Doc, but I'b afraid by case was too tough for you."

"Guess so. Well, good luck — Wait! You said *four* hours?"

"Yup. Od the buttid."

"No wonder. I'm afraid I made a terrible mistake."

"That's OK. I dod expect a coudry boy like you to haddle a case like bide. Doe hard feelings."

"I forgot to take account of all your other pills. Let's see, with Dripstop, three antibiotics, and Motrin, that should be . . . four hours and seven minutes. By my calculation, you should be clearing up just about now. Take a sniff." A muffled *shonk* emitted from the other end. "That, Anatoli, is the sound of a cold on the run. Try again."

Several seconds of silence were terminated by an exclamation. "You're right. I can breathe again. And my throat — Cut! Roll 'em! — It's perfect. Wow! I've heard people talk about these old country doctors who could cure a man just by looking at him, but I never believed — Doc, from here on, you're my main man. Name your price. I'm signing you on with the show."

"I'm honored, Anatoli, but I'll have to say no. I'm just a simple country doctor. I could never make it in show biz, I'd be like a fish out of water."

"Well . . . maybe you could script a couple of those pills on me. For the road, you know."

"I'm afraid not. If you want Green Pills, you've got to come to me."

"You're a tough man, Doc. But if that's the way you want it, it's there I go."

"I'll be here."

"Adiós, Doc. I'll see you when the faucet drips."

"Good-bye, Anatoli. Take care of yourself."

I had done it. For twenty years I had held out, steadfastly resisting temptation after temptation. There had been plenty of near misses, but always, at the last moment, I had dredged up some pharmacological justification that, however flimsy, allowed me to pretend that I was still practicing medicine as I had been trained to do, according to the principles of science and reason. But this time there could be no pretending. I had succumbed. The pills I had given Anatoli were completely worthless. It was quackery, pure and simple. The kind of thing Doc Franklin would have done without a second thought. I ought to have been ashamed. I ought to have been mortified. And yet . . .

When Maggie came into my office ten minutes later, I was staring at the wall, the receiver still resting in my right hand.

"Mrs. Blackington is ready to — Dr. Conger?"

"Huh? Sorry, Maggie. I guess I lost track of the time. I'll be there in a minute. Tell Mrs. Blackington not to worry. Tell her Dr. Conger is on her case. Good Old Doctor Conger."

"I will tell her. Are you all right, Dr. Conger?"

"Couldn't be better, Maggie. Couldn't be better."